Values-Based Commissioning of Health and Social Care

VALUES-BASED PRACTICE is a series from Cambridge University Press on values and values-based practice in medicine. Edited by Bill Fulford and Ed Peile, volumes in the series will speak to clinicians, policy makers, managers, patients and carers.

Other volumes in this new series include:

Essential Values-Based Practice: Fulford, Peile and Carroll
ISBN: 9780521530255
Values-Based Interprofessional Collaborative Practice: Thistlethwaite
ISBN: 9781107636163

Values-Based Commissioning of Health and Social Care

Christopher Heginbotham OBE
Honorary Professor, Institute of Clinical Education, Medical School,
Warwick University, Warwick, UK.

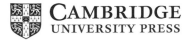

CAMBRIDGE UNIVERSITY PRESS
Cambridge, New York, Melbourne, Madrid, Cape Town,
Singapore, São Paulo, Delhi, Mexico City

Cambridge University Press
The Edinburgh Building, Cambridge CB2 8RU, UK

Published in the United States of America by Cambridge University Press, New York

www.cambridge.org
Information on this title: www.cambridge.org/9781107603356

First published 2012

Printed in the United Kingdom at the University Press, Cambridge

A catalogue record for this publication is available from the British Library

ISBN 978-1-107-60335-6 Paperback

Contents

Acknowledgements

Over the years I have worked with some excellent teachers and colleagues, but none more so than Bill Fulford and Ed Peile. Their commitment and clear-sighted approach to values-based practice has been an inspiration, and their help and support as series editors has been invaluable. I would like also to thank colleagues at Cambridge University Press for their thoughtful and helpful approach, in particular Richard Marley, Commissioning Editor, and his colleagues.

Others who have contributed or assisted in one way or another include Karen Newbigging, without whom the book would not have been possible, and a number of people who assisted with the commissioning programme that I ran with Karen at the University of Central Lancashire: Christian Dingwall, Hempsons, for his challenging ideas; Dr Louise Edwards for valuable discussions over a long period of time; Dr Jim Gardner, who encouraged me to prepare a report that became the basis of Chapter 8; Andrew Jackson and Bryn Shorney, for their support with information management for commissioning; Professor Antony Sheehan, for his prescient approach to commissioning; Dr Michael Taylor for invaluable clinical insights; Nigel Walker, who taught on the course and contributed many policy ideas; and Professor Eric Wolstenholme, David Monk, and colleagues at *symmetric* who offered advice on whole-systems thinking and modelling. I must also express a real debt of gratitude to all the students who took one of the University of Central Lancashire postgraduate certificates in commissioning for helpful and often challenging debates.

Finally, I must thank my wife, also Chris, for her forbearance over the summer 2011 when I did almost nothing else but write; and our four daughters, Emily, Sarah, Laura, and Elizabeth, who are a constant delight and inspiration. As always I remain responsible for any omissions or inaccuracies.

I wish to acknowledge the following permissions:

Professor B. Haynes and the *British Medical Journal* for permission to use diagram 8 from Haynes *et al.* (2002).

Professor Michael Porter for permission to use the Five Forces diagram (Diagrams 32 and 33) from Competitive Advantage (Porter, 1985).

The Office for National Statistics for permission to use the graphs 16 and 17 under the Open Government Licence v. 10.

The UK Department of Health for permission to use the Spearhead Group graphics at Diagrams 18 and 19 under the Open Government Licence v. 10; and Diagram 20: 'Connected ecosystem of health and social systems' (*Source*: Dr Jo Nurse, New Horizons Programme).

Preface: Values-based Commissioning

Values-based practice is not another category of commissioning to rank with practice-based commissioning, locality commissioning, or commissioning for outcomes in health and social care. Values-basing is about the processes that can be applied to any form of commissioning, anywhere. This book explores these processes. The UK revolution in commissioning health and social care makes a very convenient backdrop, but not a reason, for a highly topical discussion of what values-basing really means.

Values-based commissioning describes the theoretical and practical demands on clinicians and social care professionals of using stated values to achieve an improved process for filtering the available evidence to achieve improved outcomes for patients and service users. Commissioning is a complex and iterative process that requires commissioners to balance evidence and values so as to achieve the best health and social care appropriate to the needs of individuals.

Health and social care commissioning is a values-driven as well as evidence-driven enterprise. Although there has increasingly been an expectation that the evidence base of commissioning should be made fully explicit, the corresponding values base has by and large been left largely implicit. Values-based commissioning thus complements evidence-based commissioning by providing a skills base and other support processes for working with differences of values that are held by all those engaged in making commissioning decisions.

This book describes the challenge of values-based commissioning (V-BC). For some, that challenge is theoretical – why should V-BC improve the way we commission care, and how will values help? Others will be concerned that there are insufficient resources needed to engage patients and service users regularly in a truly satisfactory way; for yet others, it is not so much their commitment that is in question as the pressure on the health service at a time of severe restraint. There is no doubt the austerity programmes that affect everyone but especially the UK and the USA during 2011–2012 have taken their toll. However, V-BC should not be optional. It should be complementary to evidence-based practice (E-BP)[1] at all times.

What are values? The first thing to say is that the discussion in the book is not too arduous philosophically. That is not to say we should not be rigorous, but there is a lengthy debate to be had, separately, about the role of values, preferences, beliefs and desires, their differences, and their relevance to health and social care, although that is in part covered in Fulford *et al.* (2012, forthcoming), in the same book series. Are some values virtues? Or should values and virtues be kept separate? Are some beliefs values? While, for example, religious beliefs may not be to everyone's liking, they are often strongly held and shape some people's values. Are some desires values? Or are values the consequences, or conversely perhaps, the antecedents of our desires? We are not so much concerned here with what *should* be considered a value, but what *is* practically a value that must be taken into account. In the debate on abortion, for example, there are differing and strongly held values on either side of the argument. To recognise that fact does not necessarily require us to enter the debate about abortion per se!

---

[1] We will use the term evidence-based practice (E-BP) throughout rather than evidence-based medicine (E-BM) except where the latter is directly appropriate; and we will use the term values-based commissioning (V-BC) except where values-based practice (V-BP) has a more generic feel.

The challenge of V-BC is fourfold. First, there are many values some of which are not usually engaged in health and social care, although they may be part of the wider culture from which patients and service users are drawn. Understanding those values is necessary to ensure that everyone and especially minority groups and cultures are given due weight in all health and social care discussions. Second, values can be written in various ways, but are usually normative statements that affirm how things should be or ought to be, which things are good or bad, or which actions are right or wrong. Values are the principles with which we lead our lives; some are held more firmly than others, but everyone has them!

Third, 'values' cover many aspects of life which impinge peripherally on health and social care; these may not be our most pressing concerns, but sometimes they become much more important for short periods or for small but significant matters. For example, my childcare arrangements may have very little to do with my health care demands; but if the clinic appointment happens to coincide with my caring duties, to which I am committed, the clash may take on more important character at that moment. Fourth, values concern the felt aspects of illness, as opposed to the factual issues of disease; values are an essential component of any serious discussion about health and social care.

Values-based commissioning is thus the reflection of our values in a discussion of the evidence. In Chapter 1 we will note that V-BC seeks a full understanding of recognised individual, group, community and population values with which to develop a picture of the community in relation to a particular health or social care matter. This is then used creatively and comprehensively to reflect the evidence base and to determine the best way to offer care, giving due weight to the values as expressed. As we shall see in Chapter 2, there are many differing values that can be engaged, and the NHS, public health, well-being, and social care reforms demonstrate how important values are.

Chapter 3 is a discussion of the government's reform programme. Whether this will become law, and if it does, how it will be implemented and the problems and opportunities it may bring, are at once of interest in providing the present context *and* irrelevant to effective values-based practice. V-BC is an essential component of health and social care commissioning independent of the current legislative, organisational or policy driven structure of the NHS and local authorities. Readers may wish to skip the discussion if they feel they have sufficient understanding of the government's intentions; or conversely, they may find the discussion of the context illuminating.

Chapter 4 then considers evidence and outcomes, identifying the 'other side of the coin' – evidence-based practice, and the way that E-BP and V-BP (values-based practice) interact. V-BP enables commissioners to identify and make explicit the often diverse values of all those engaged in the process of commissioning, and to map those values onto a carefully prepared framework (Fulford *et al.*, 2012, forthcoming). By drawing on the diversity of values so far identified – Chapter 5 considers the role of community and public engagement in obtaining values – commissioners then have a resource for balanced decision-making within the context defined by the framework. The framework can then be used to engage with a continuing process of evidence-based review, bringing personal, community and professional values into contention with the qualitative and quantitative evidence drawn from the scientific (social, physical and psychological) research literature.

Chapter 6 considers values in public health, especially in relation to enhanced morbidity and mortality from deprivation, and 'prior discriminations' suffered by minority communities. The social determinants of health are often given a specific twist as a result of discrimination by society or individual institutions. Chapter 7 then takes health and social care together. Integrative commissioning demands a V-BC approach that seeks to link the values of the NHS and social care, patients and clients, clinicians and social care staff. Integrative suggests and anticipates actual integration. We do not need to have wholly integrated systems to pursue an integrative strategy.

Values go wider and deeper than ethics. Values are explicit in some areas of medicine, as we shall see in Chapter 8 on priority setting when we discuss cost–benefit and cost–utility analyses that form the basis of health (and increasingly social care) guidelines (Brown *et al.*, 2005). Existing resources for values-based practice include decision theory, health economics, social science and the medical humanities (Fulford *et al.*, 2002).

Chapter 9 addresses outcomes and the perennial problem of describing an outcome in terms that make it measurable, attractive to policy makers, appropriate for contracts, and meaningful for patients and service users. Chapter 10 takes a long look at market stimulation and market ideology, identifying the appropriate role of the private sector and demonstrating the importance of social enterprise and the third sector. Finally, Chapter 11 considers management and leadership of health and social care. A carefully focussed discussion of the literature on leadership demonstrates that values are indeed inherent to the whole enterprise

Values-based commissioning is the practice of recognising and acting on the differing values held by all those engaged in making health and social care decisions, in order to plan and implement health and social care that is culturally relevant and appropriate, clinically and economically effective, and addresses need in a way that reflects the values of those using and providing care. This in turn requires commissioners to hold a commitment to make explicit their values as well as those of local communities, patients and service users (Jensen and Mooney, 1990; Woodbridge and Fulford, 2004).

The book is embedded primarily in the experience of the UK, particularly England. However, its message applies just as much to other jurisdictions, notably the Anglophone countries (such as Australia, Canada and the USA). For example, the discussion in Chapter 1 on the derivation and deliberation about values and in Chapter 4 on evidence and outcomes apply as much to other countries as to England. Market ideology will appeal to countries with a large private sector, as will Chapter 11, which draws heavily on the US literature. Soundings taken with clinicians in the USA suggest that the theme of this book will have a ready audience, especially among clinicians and medical managers who want to achieve improvements (and cost savings) that are acceptable to patients.

Overall, values-based commissioning reflects not a programmatic approach to commissioning, such as locality commissioning or practice-based commissioning. Rather, it reflects a fundamental need to understand the values of the people served in whatever way commissioning is undertaken. The book will appeal to commissioners of whatever stripe as they struggle with governments' change programmes at a time of austerity. Values-based practice will help to achieve a better and more responsive health and social care programme acceptable to all patients and service users.

Christopher Heginbotham
Priest Hutton

Abbreviations

3Is	Institute for Innovation and Improvement		JSNA	joint strategic needs assessment
ADL	activities of daily living		LA	Local Authority
APHO	Association of Public Health Observatories		LE	life expectancy
			MCDA	multi-criteria decision analysis
ASCOT	Adult Social Care Outcomes Toolkit		MDS	minimum data set
			MoH	Medical Officer of Health
BME	Black and minority ethnic		MOPSU	Measuring Outcomes for Public Service Users
CABG	Coronary Artery Bypass Graft		MSOA	Middle Level Super Output Area
CBA	cost–benefit analysis		NEET	not in education, employment or training
CBT	cognitive-behavioural therapy			
CCG	Clinical Commissioning Group		NIESR	National Institute of Economic and Social research
CCP	Cooperation and Competition Panel			
			NIMHE	National Institute for Mental Health, England
CEA	cost-effectiveness analysis			
CHD	coronary heart disease		OFT	Office for Fair Trading
CIP	Percutaneous Coronary Intervention		PbC	practice-based commissioning
			PBMA	Programme Budgeting and Marginal Analysis
CQUIN	Commissioning for Quality and Innovation			
			PbR	payment by results
CUA	cost–utility analysis		PCT	primary care trust
DALYs	Disability Adjusted Life Years		PRCC	Principles and Rules of Cooperation and Competition
DCLG	Department for Communities and Local Government			
			PSA	Public Service Agreement
DFLE	disability-free life expectancy		QALYs	Quality Adjusted Life Years
DH	Department of Health		QIPP	Quality, Innovation, Productivity and Prevention
DMU	directly managed unit			
E-BM	evidence-based medicine		QOF	Quality and Outcomes Framework
E-BP	evidence-based practice			
ECHR	the European Convention on Human Rights		RCT	randomised controlled trial
			SHA	Strategic Health Authority
FOIA	Freedom of Information Act		SII	slope index of inequality
GP	general practitioner		TPP	total purchasing pilot
GPCC	GP Commissioning Consortia		UA	Unitary Authority
H&WB	Health and Well-being Board		UDHR	Universal Declaration on Human Rights
HAQ-DI	Health Assessment Questionnaire Disability Index			
			V-BC	values-based commissioning
HLE	healthy life expectancy		V-BP	values-based practice
IB	individual budgets		VFM	value for money
IM	infant mortality		VM	values matrix
IPU	individual practice unit		WCC	World Class Commissioning

Chapter

1

Values-based practice in health and social care

Purpose and scope

This book is intended to assist all those charged with commissioning health and social care in the UK and in other jurisdictions that have similar organisational arrangements. The term 'values-based commissioning' begs for definitions. These are discussed in some detail in this chapter and elsewhere. At this point it is worth clarifying the broad purpose and scope of the book.

Commissioning is a complex, iterative process that ensures that health and social care provision for a population is clinically and cost-effective and appropriate to the needs of the people for whom it is intended. Commissioning is not simply planning or procurement. Commissioning has a number of stages described in different ways by various authors, and in different countries and jurisdictions, but all contain something along the following lines.

Commissioning has a cyclical form that begins with assessing the health and social care needs in the communities served; consults and involves patients and the public alongside community, patients and service user organisations; defines the care outcomes appropriate to the population served; identifies the types of interventions (medical, surgical, social or psychological) that may be appropriate to the conditions to be treated or ameliorated; gathers information on all those providers that may be able to or wish to contribute a component of the care pathway (subject to some over-arching policy on the use of NHS providers); invests in capacity-building organisations to provide tailored and effective care; encourages all reasonable providers to become involved through ensuring that contracting processes are fair and transparent; develops acceptable risk-sharing arrangements; and establishes feedback processes that catalyse further innovation and engagement of patients and the public.

Each of the nested clauses in the previous paragraph can be 'unpacked' and are considered in much greater detail in the following chapters. It can be seen at once that commissioning is not simply a matter of contracting or procurement. It is rather a process of needs determination and then finding the best, most cost- and clinically or professionally effective solution. This may mean using existing NHS or local authority services, or it may require community groups to be encouraged to offer culturally relevant and appropriate solutions to local needs. It may mean using the private sector, or third-sector organisations that are increasingly important partners in offering tailor-made personalised care for specific needs within those communities. Social enterprises offer alternative prescriptions. The challenge is to balance the needs of the majority, and thus the cost-effectiveness of care with offering person-centred services that address individual need.

Values-based commissioning

If commissioning is a complex and iterative process, what do we mean by 'values-based' commissioning? Health and social care commissioning is a values-driven as well as an evidence-driven enterprise. However, whereas there has increasingly been an expectation that the evidence base of commissioning should be made fully explicit, the corresponding values base has by and large been left largely implicit. Values-based commissioning thus complements evidence-based commissioning by providing a skills base and other support processes for working with differences of values that are held by all those engaged in making commissioning decisions.

It should be obvious that, if (for the moment) the definition of commissioning given above is accepted without argument, it raises a number of important questions about 'how we know what we know' and the basis for making judgements about what we are told or learn from the processes described. For example, as commissioners, how do we decide that a 'need' is something that we should consider our responsibility to do something about, or to ignore, or to find a non-NHS or health care response?

We are immediately in the familiar, albeit still far from straightforward, territory of deciding whether this 'need' should be met. Is this normative need (for example, something that medicine might consider a standard condition-treatment option); is it required in comparison to those who do have this 'need' (for example, in relation to health inequalities); is it a 'felt need' from the perspective of the person who claims that need; or an 'expressed need' which may or may not be a 'want' rather than a necessity (Bradshaw, 1972)?[1] We can only really get to the root of these linked questions if we consider carefully not only the (objective) evidence base for the need (for example, epidemiological evidence) but also the reasons why people feel or express their need. In other words, the values that they hold and which they bring to any discussion about need. As Jane Hirshfield put it, '[W]e are psychologically made visible by our desires' (Hirshfield, 2008, p. 21).

Values-based practice enables commissioners to identify and make explicit the often very diverse values of all those involved whether as commissioners, as providers or as users of services. This diversity can then be mapped onto an explicit, carefully prepared framework that includes not only ethical values but also the needs, wishes, aspirations, strengths and resources of the services, the community and individuals. By drawing on the diversity of values so far identified, commissioners then have a resource for balanced decision-making within the context defined by the framework, which is why the way that framework is defined is so crucial. The framework can then be used to engage with an continuing process of evidence-based review, bringing personal, community and professional values into contention with the qualitative and quantitative evidence drawn from the scientific (social, physical and psychological) research literature. Fulford *et al.* (2012, forthcoming) describe the framework and process in detail.

Values go wider and deeper than ethics. By patient values we mean the unique preferences, concerns and expectations each patient brings to the clinical encounter and which must be integrated into clinical decisions if they are to service the patient. The common feature of values, which is what makes them directly relevant to medical decision-making, is that they are 'prescriptive' or 'action guiding' (Hare, 1952). So values are explicit in some

---

[1] Bradshaw (1972) described these four types of need in a now classic paper that has been referred to frequently over the years.

areas of medicine, as we shall see in Chapter 8 on priority setting, when we discuss cost–benefit and cost–utility analyses that form the basis of health (and increasingly social care) guidelines (Brown *et al.*, 2005). Existing resources for values-based practice include decision theory, health economics, social science and the medical humanities (Fulford *et al.*, 2002).

Current policy priorities driving the need for values-based as well as evidence-based commissioning include primary care-led (perhaps better described as clinician-led commissioning, in which commissioners will have to engage with widely divergent cultural values), integrative commissioning of health and social care that recognises the special contribution of families and communities, and the personalisation of services (the basis of which is individually defined needs). Values-based commissioning is effective in such contexts not because it allows everyone's expectations to be satisfied, but because it provides a process that is seen to be transparent, fair and balanced. Values-based commissioning is successful to the extent that everyone feels their voice has been heard.

It will by now be apparent that values-based commissioning is the practice of recognising and acting on the differing values held by all those engaged in making health and social care decisions, in order to plan and implement health and social care that is culturally relevant and appropriate, clinically and economically effective, and addresses need in a way that reflects the values of those using and providing care. This in turn requires commissioners to make explicit their values as well as those of local communities, patients and service users (Jensen and Mooney, 1990; Woodbridge and Fulford, 2004).

Values differences

The values that people hold differ enormously: what may be important to one person may be of little significance to another. V-BC provides a framework for commissioners and commissioning practice that recognises the diversity and multiplicity of values, and raises awareness of the way values relate, interact and impact on experiences, actions and relationships in health and social care commissioning. Sometimes values are seen as synonymous with ethics. However, values are much wider than ethical principles even though ethical considerations matter greatly in health and social care. Values cover what is valued by all those who commission or use health services. This includes not only ethical values (or principles) – justice, best interests, not doing harm, autonomy – but also wishes, desires, beliefs, ideals, or needs, in addition to ideas on quality of life, self-fulfilment, flourishing, and well-being (Woodbridge and Fulford, 2004).

V-BC draws on the insights of V-BP, which identifies differences in values as crucial to effective clinical and professional practice (Woodbridge and Fulford, 2004). Clinical, social and organisational values differ between professional groups, commissioning organisations, patients, service users and the general public. Where values are common, there is less likely to be disagreement about decisions on health and social care provision; where values differ, there is an opportunity to debate those differences and use the debate to focus on possibly contentious matters that require resolution before complex, challenging and difficult decisions can be taken. Where values conflict, there is an opportunity for learning, for sharing the reasons for those differences, for greater understanding, and for achieving a resolution acceptable to all parties.

The practice of medicine, health and social care is *always* values-driven, even if those values are not made explicit. Decisions on allocating resources to services, or individual treatments, are not value-free. Often, the values that underpin a public service are those of a dominant professional or cultural group; sometimes they are informed by individual concerns and prejudice; sometimes they are enforced by and embedded within legislation. V-BC provides a powerful context for commissioning health and social care, where the values of clinicians, managers, organisations, patients and service users may differ. V-BC recognises diversity and difference and emphasises the importance of making values explicit in order to highlight differences in the ways that patients and service users can expect to be treated. Real and effective commissioning (and, for that matter, de-commissioning) can only be achieved through an authentic understanding of the values held by the community.

While some values are universal (such as the right to life, or freedom from torture or degrading treatment), even these values can be contentious in health care. The right to life cannot be considered a right to be kept alive at any cost. V-BC catalyses a debate about the values to adopt in any culture or community when making decisions about the most appropriate forms of treatment, care or support to offer a patient or family.

Values-based commissioning encourages recognition of diversity and difference – by income level, ethnicity, age, gender, disability, faith and sexuality – and through differing perspectives or cultures, personal motivations, strongly held beliefs (religious, cultural, political, or familial). Values may differ but individuals often hold coherent albeit complex, and over-lapping, value sets. Values are not static. Differing values may not indicate competing interpretations but complementary aspects of a highly complex concept. They vary over time and place for individuals and communities. What is considered right at one time or place may be thought wrong at another. VBC requires robust processes of community and individual engagement that go beyond tentative public involvement strategies. True engagement places communities centrally in the commissioning process working as genuine partners with professional staff and commissioning organisations.

Shared decision-making

Values-based commissioning is not the same as shared decision-making. The latter is an important part of provider-side practice that enables patients and service users to become involved in decisions about their care in a well-informed way. Shared decision-making is a process 'in which clinicians and patients work together to select tests, treatments, management or support packages, based on clinical evidence and the patient's informed preferences.' It involves 'evidence based information about options, outcomes and uncertainties . . . with decision support counselling and . . . recording' (Coulter and Collins, 2011). The emphasis on evidence in this definition suggests that this is one half of the field, that of evidence. Shared decision-making enables that part of the equation to be made real. However, it does little to ensure that patients' values are understood or used in the determination of treatments. This is acknowledged in the breach, so to speak, by Coulter and Collins in the way they describe shared decision-making always as 'preferences' and never as 'values'. Preferences flow from understanding the evidence; values from inner beliefs and motivations.

There is good evidence from a number of studies that patients and service users who are fully engaged in decisions about health and social care have better outcomes. The distinction between shared decision-making, self-management support and personalised care planning is that they have similar philosophies rooted in a concern to use the evidence as wisely as possible. What matters are the practical nuts and bolts of self-management and care planning rather than the underlying attitudes and values that are brought to the table. Patients and service users want more information in a clear and simple, jargon-free manner. It must be available immediately and at all stages of the patients' and service users' care and treatment pathway. Using the evidence and information as decision aids or recognition of decision points in the pathway is a valuable approach to evidence. What is then required is a structured values-based process that builds on the mechanisms of care (the disease element) to add the human element (the feelings of illness or well-being).

The growing complexity of values in health and social care is due to a number of factors, some that are general to society as a whole and some specific to medicine or social work, health sciences (such as epidemiology) or social sciences (such as cultural studies). Progressively, patients and families are engaged more in decision-making with clinicians ('voice and choice'); the increasingly wide treatment options created by advances in science and technology are strongly value-laden. Multi-disciplinary teamwork suggests that there is no one dominant narrative, which necessitates all professions to have their say (Fulford *et al.*, 2002).

Fact-value distinction

Not everyone agrees with the desirability or acceptability of fact and value (e.g. Putnam, 2002). An ordinary 'distinction' between fact and value does not have only one meaning – it is not unambiguous. We can have a range of differing interpretations depending on the partitioning of the values space, and the nature of the value judgements. On the other hand, a 'dichotomy' presupposes a division into two parts or categories, particularly when they are acutely differentiated or divergent. In our scheme, fact and value are not so sharply distinguished. Indeed, fact and value are entangled to a noteworthy extent and derive part of their meaning from each other. Scientific research depends on values; values are shaped by evidence. Much of our descriptive language confronts notions of 'fact' and 'ought to shake the confidence of anyone that there is a notion of *fact* that contrasts neatly . . . with the notion of "value" supposedly invoked in . . . "value judgements"' (Putnam, 2002, p. 26).

Values are used to describe 'qualities that guide our actions and subject our (human) activities to be worthy of praise or blame' (Sadler, 2004). They are not context-free: a decision on whether to treat a statement as implying a value judgement depends significantly on context and the way that enables an interpretation. 'Thick' value terms also 'exhibit a complex mix of factually descriptive and evaluatively descriptive meanings' (Sadler, 2004, p. 31), which must be considered carefully in actual practice. Similarly, there may be value-related consequences to particular choices within a theory or classification.

Values come in many sizes and shapes. Epistemic values are related to rationality and are concerned directly with evaluation of scientific theory (see above the idea of 'entanglement', and in Chapter 4 on rationality); this contains words such as coherence, precision or simplicity. Ethical values are those pertaining to moral or immoral conduct, using words such as autonomy, beneficence, malfeasance or justice. Pragmatic or utilitarian values concern the economic or efficient use of resources, with terms such as well-organised, competent or cooperative. Ontological values are highly relevant to the self and to ideas of time and causality; they are 'deeply presupposed' (Sadler, 2004, p. 38) and because of this are relevant to psychiatric disorders especially. Finally, aesthetic values are those that tell us something about beauty and proportion, but may also include 'economical' and 'resourceful' where those terms are affective rather than pragmatic. This is not a hard and fast taxonomy, but rather a description that suggests ways of viewing values and their use in practice.

When we use values, particularly in determining the right way to provide care, or in obtaining a population perspective on a service, the words we use offer a clue to the appropriate way to behave and deal with the presenting problem. This will be especially true in challenging the available evidence with a set of epistemic beliefs about the underlying science or in deciding that a study was not undertaken ethically, for whatever reason. More importantly, both for groups and individuals, ontological values will be brought into play. Where a concept is highly contentious (for example, community treatment orders in psychiatry) then these concepts will be important precursors to understanding the correct way to use the evidence in the light of an individual's set of principles, beliefs, aspirations, hope and goals. Indeed, values-based practice is based on theoretical work undertaken in analytic philosophy concerned with the meanings and implications of value terms (Fulford, 1989).

One set of values that we have not touched on are spiritual and personal values. Spiritual traditions challenge the self-centred and material culture, but 'offer an alternative system of values-based on selflessness, compassion and wisdom' (Rubin, 2007, p. 147). Being poor is not a virtue, but affluence does not resolve fundamental emotional and spiritual problems. 'A world of timeless egos adopting and discarding styles of self-presentation and self-assertion, is a social as well as philosophical shambles' (Williams, 2000, p. 49). Ontological values will thus include those that apply to particular cultures and communities. In the West there is, compared to many cultures in other countries, an astonishing degree of individualism (Conway, 2007). Whether smart men in the city dressed in suits, or the young teenagers with expensive trainers and hoodies, each is a tendency to re-establish a tribe of sorts. Conversely, the tribal nature of societies as far apart as Libya or Pakistan provide a different way of interpreting values with collective agreements that may tend to conservatism but with a degree of coherence. The multi-cultural and multi-ethnic society demands that we recognise differing and diverse values in deciding on the evidence we use and the care we give.

Ten principles of values-based practice

Commissioning health and social care includes the functions of identifying need, determining ways of meeting that need, engaging with patients and service users, negotiating with providers or suppliers, capacity-building local organisations and communities, and making decisions on which services, at what quality and in what quantity to fund. The current and continuing emphasis on personalisation demands recognition of the differing values held by recipients of personalised care packages. As health and social care moves inexorably towards individual health or social budgets, V-BC will be a necessary underpinning of the process of determining the financial and service response.

Values-based commissioning is the essential requirement of acceptable and legitimate health and social care development. Focusing on the values of all those involved in determining the most appropriate health and social care for a community will ensure the widest acceptance and legitimacy of the increasingly tough decisions required. One reason for this is the distinction between the value of health (value-in-use), and the value of health care (value-in-exchange) (Mooney and McGuire, 1988, p. 7). It is 'only the consumer/patient who can attach a value-in-use to health status' (Mooney and McGuire, 1988). In other words, the outcomes of care can only really be known to the patient. The treating clinicians will have an informed view, but the feelings as well as the evidence can be assessed fully by the patient alone, but with some help and support.

As we have seen, V-BP aims to support balanced decision-making within a framework of shared-values practice based on mutual respect and relying for its practical effectiveness on good process rather than pre-set right outcomes (Fulford *et al.*, 2012, forthcoming). Values will usually be in tension or conflict, and V-BP provides the skills and other resources for balanced decision-making in individual cases. However, what about the case of groups or communities? How do we use V-BP for making priority decisions or resource allocation between conflicting groups with differing values?

First, of course, we must recognise that V-BP and its sister, evidence-based medicine (or practice; E-BP) are two sides of the same coin. As Fulford *et al.* (2012, forthcoming) suggest, V-BP and E-BP must be carefully weighed and made reciprocal. They quote the National Institute for Mental Health, England (NIMHE) Values Framework which is itself based on two parts: a first half that provides an important guide to NIMHE's work, and a second part that sets out those values held to be of especial importance to NIMHE and mental health service development. The first half is three R's of V-BP: recognition, raising awareness, and respect. 'Recognition' is concerned with the proper balance of evidence and values; raising awareness concerns diversity; and respect is a direct reference to the basis of V-BP as a foundational programme. 'Recognition' goes beyond the importance of noting and acting on both values and evidence, towards, as we will see in Chapter 5, a recognition and acceptance of diversity and difference.

The 10 principles of V-BP demonstrate that, as so often, it is good process that makes for good decisions (Fulford, 2004). They are:

- four principles of clinical skills,
- two principles of relationships,
- three principles of science and values together, and
- a final important principle: 'dissensus'.

The four principles of clinical skills are:

- awareness of values – the importance of accepting and addressing the tension and possible conflict of values;
- reasoning – about values and evidence, with patients or service users, and understanding their views, aspirations, background, culture and information;
- knowledge – recognising that values are important even to someone who a professional person might consider to be 'beyond the pale', such as a heavy smoker with cancer but who refuses to quit smoking; and
- communication skills – perhaps a crucial and obvious requirement of values-based practice.

The two principles about relationships are concerned with the quality of professional relationships with service users, and thus cover:

- person-centred care, which is determined by and contributes to values-based practice; and
- multi-disciplinary practices and teamwork, which includes all those who have a locus in the process.

The further three principles are practical and may be 'red flags' in the process (Fulford *et al.*, 2012, forthcoming).

- The two-feet principle recognises that all decisions are based on the two feet of evidence and values. If a problem seems to be no more than checking or establishing the facts then there is probably a difficulty with values.

- The squeaky-wheel principle suggests that we notice values when they become problematic. In fact this is one of those principles that is important because it sums up the core issue at the heart of V-BP – that it is where values are in tension that the work gets done. As Fulford *et al.* (2012) suggest, however, this also 'flags' for us that, most likely, if the problem appears to be one only of values, then we may have missed something to do with the evidence.

- The science-driven principle draws attention to the importance of both facts and values together, and suggests that especially, although not exclusively, for hi-tech medicine it is essential to look out for hidden facts and values.

Finally, the tenth principle is 'dissensus' (Fulford, 2011b). Dissensus is 'agreeing to disagree', an outcome that is peculiar to values-based practice. Undertaking values-based commissioning requires that clinical commissioners (general practitioners (GPs), nurses, hospital doctors, etc.), patients and service users and their families, and the community in various guises, are all involved in the process. However, at the end of the day, not all values can be brought into the equation. Some values may be held over, not discarded but retained to be balanced by another subject on another day. There is no harm in this, if everyone accepts the process, which must of course be seen to be fair, open, transparent and honest.

Facts and values

While we have little space to go into details about the reasons for facts and values, there is no doubt that the history of this process is filled with attempts to dismantle the edifice created. More importantly, the divide between facts and values has a long and credible history, especially the idea that a value can be constructed from a fact (rather than vice versa). Hume (2000) noted that arguments often proceed by making factual statements only to end with a conclusion about values. To Hume this was 'altogether inconceivable'. Similarly, Moore (1903, reprinted 2000) suggested that it is a 'mistake to analyse an ethical statement by defining good in a way that points to any natural property' (described in Orr, 2011). For almost 300 years there has been an austere discouragement for the idea that facts and values might be related too closely.

There are those, as we have seen, who believe that the distinction has no (or little) reasonable basis (Putnam, 2002). However, by and large, the difference is not only useful, but essential to a proper analysis of why we do things in the way we do. More importantly it is the range and nature of facts and values that provides the opportunity to develop a process of priority-setting and resource allocation. Fulford (2011a) has shown that the practice of evidence-based and values-based practice are two halves of the same field. On the one half is disease – a set of facts – and these 'cash out' as a failure of function (of the body). So, if deterioration occurs, caused by something such as renal disease, then the failure that results is loss of renal function. This is the consequence of focusing on fact. The fact of the disease leads to a failure of some bodily function. The other half of the field is 'illness', an evaluative not a factual term. This 'cashes out', as Bill Fulford describes it, as failure of 'action'. An illness is a 'feeling' of being ill, a term that identifies the person as 'under the weather'. A person may feel ill and may or may not be diseased, or at least not seriously. Conversely, having a 'disease' denotes a bacterium or a virus that can be cultured, or a tumour or other lesion, and does not necessarily mean you feel 'ill'.

That is all very well for a bacterium or a virus, but what do we say to a disease such as coronary heart disease or, rather differently, a broken leg. The former is based on diagnostic tests that can show the presence of narrowed arteries – a fact; the latter is, of course, by

Table 1.1 Facts and values.

	Facts	Overlap (entanglement)	Values
No disease	No disease entity	Challenges to the way disease is measured	Feeling of illness
Disease	Disease entity such as evidence of a bacterium or virus	Challenges to the way feelings are described	May not feel ill but may have latent disease

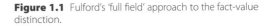

Figure 1.1 Fulford's 'full field' approach to the fact-value distinction.

definition a 'fact'. These situations may still make the person feel unwell, and indeed may be serious, but they have a definite basis in fact. More difficult are those situations where I may have a serious illness but do know it. An early cancerous growth may not manifest for months or years, and in the meantime I feel well even though I have a serious disease. On the other hand, I may feel ill as a result of drinking too much alcohol the night before, but I do not have a disease (assuming I am not an alcoholic or suffering from a hepatic disorder). See Figure 1.1.

The importance of values-based practice is that it recognises the interplay of the two sets of data, the factual and the evaluative. The 'full field' approach thus generated provides a number of opportunities. In the first place it suggests that the two halves of the field overlap and that a number of insights emerge at the intersection that is generated. These can be represented by Table 1.1.

Second, in some cases (for example, mental illness) we can consider other elements such as capacity to consent or refuse treatment. The term 'action' suggests 'agency', an ability to make decisions for oneself. This may be affected, to the extent of attenuating the person's decision-making responses, by a feeling of illness even if there is no evident disease entity. Conversely, the effect of a proven disease may not have the necessary implications of reducing the ability to make a decision. Indeed, this distinction has caused untold difficulties with patients over the years.

Third, being 'ill' may be a smokescreen to hide behind when there is no disease present. 'I feel ill' has been used for centuries as an exculpating reason not to do something. This can be useful 'in the limit', but does not assist us in devising an effective values-based practice.

Values-based commissioning thus reinforces the desire to identify disease (or its equivalent in social care) from the feelings of illness where there is no disease present. As we have seen, 'feeling ill' translates into a failure of action, either deliberately or involuntarily; being 'diseased' requires some form of care, although that may be relatively simple, such as offering personal pastoral support. It is here that we come to the crux of the full field system. It does not suggest that health deals with treatment, and social care with evaluative positions. Rather social care and health both have factual and evaluative dimensions.

Table 1.2 The interplay between the fact–value distinction and health and social care.

	Health	Social care
Facts	Identifiable disease entity or other factual description	Lack of aids to daily living (money, housing, transport, etc.) ('I cannot cope because . . .')
Values	Illness or other feeling that may or may not require intervention	Needs assessment (normative, comparative, felt, expressed) ('I feel unable to cope')

Table 1.3 Facts and values in relation to individual and population perspectives.

	Individual	Population
Facts (disease)	Shared decision-making	Public health
Values (illness)	Personal values-based commissioning	'Proportionate universalism'[2] based on population values

Table 1.2 also throws into relief the nature of this distinction. Facts are facts, although they may be disputed, but values often have a factual aura. In health and social care we note that the person's situation is a result of some decision(s), perhaps recent, perhaps from many years ago, that has left the person with a feeling of illness or not coping. The evidence base is often thought of as evidence-based medicine (E-BM), but must surely for these purposes be widened to evidence-based practice (E-BP); that is, both evidence of what works in medicine (an amalgam of science and human values), and in social care (an amalgam of responsible opportunities and social action).

The nature of local authority Health and Well-being Boards proposed by the government will thus grapple with a complicated mix of health and social care facts and values. It does not follow that 'health' provides E-BM and 'well-being' (or social care) offers ways in the community to address lifestyle concerns. Health (the NHS and private and voluntary companies) offer a range of evidence- *and* values-based approaches; social care offers well-being interventions alongside traditional social care, but based on an assessment of the evidence of what works (and how well it works) and the values of individuals, groups and communities. How those values are determined, and the ways in which they can be used is, the subject of Chapter 2. Health and social care resources need to be pooled and aimed in the first instance at cost–benefit-proven universal and targeted population benefits. What is left can then be used to tackle a range of values-based opportunities, some of which, but not all, will have an evidence base.

Most importantly, viewing E-BM through a values-based lens will enable evidence to be assessed by those who will be most affected. How that will be done is a matter of some conjecture, but in Chapter 7 we will offer some suggestions, especially on the way that NICE Guidelines can be used to treat patients and can be over-ridden where patients and service users have good reasons to want something else. See Table 1.3.

Values-based practice is thus implicitly tied to outcomes and to outcomes-led commissioning. As we consider the interplay of values and evidence, it becomes apparent that we must consider the outcomes that we can achieve from the interventions that we agree. If the

---

[2] We will discuss proportionate universalism in Chapter 7.

values of a person challenge the values enshrined in, say, NICE guidelines, then it is on the basis largely of outcomes that the challenge is made. There may be examples of process challenges, but these are either challenges to the detail of the process or mostly trivial in relation to the outcome desired.

Individuals, groups, community, or population

A lot of values-based medicine and healthcare is concerned with awareness of values, in particular addressing tensions and possible conflicts, and reasoning with patients or service users about their views, aspirations, backgrounds, and cultures. We do this with all the tools at our disposal, notably by listening openly, offering opportunities for patients to become full participants in a shared approach, and paying close attention to the communication strategy that we adopt. At the end, however, every discussion is about health, well-being or social care for one (or possibly a very small number) patient or service user. Commissioning considers populations, communities, or groups of patients, service users, clients, consumers, and customers. Commissioning is like epidemiology in that regard. We must recognise that we have to commission services for both individuals and populations, and it is a truism that the individuals are treated but the population benefits.

Many doctors, when first educated in epidemiology, want to retreat to the well-worn doctor–patient relationship that they were first taught. It takes a while to find their feet naturally talking about populations, about statistics, and about cohorts of patients. Similarly in social care, the individual service user or client is provided with an individual budget following assessment, but the Director of Adult Social Services needs to have a population perspective on the implications of the commissioned care. Consequently there is in this book a constant division between V-BP as practiced with individuals and that practiced with groups. V-BP with groups and communities is more difficult as we do not have the individual biography or personal values set on which to base our considerations. Conversely, grouping values together will sometimes provide stronger agreement on core values with others left to the sides. These peripheral values are not unimportant, and will need to be considered by a treating clinician, but the core agreed values offer some stability to the discussion.

Choice is a value. But what is the objective of choice(s)? It would appear to be a 'good', and the objective of shaping and determining goods is usually described as *valuing*. The goods that are the entities of *valuing* we call *values*. However, values can be intrinsic, extrinsic or systemic patterns of relative weights given to the properties of things or things in themselves. This underlines 'the relation of goods to human perceptions and choices, and to properties in and among things' (Pellegrino and Thomasma, 1988) which are fluid, continually reappraised and amended and are in a state of change. From this we can see that health itself is a value (rather than 'is valued' or 'has value'), and means that choice 'need not be limited to promoting individual good at the expense of social good or vice versa' (Pellegrino and Thomasma, 1988). Medicine and 'health' are neither of the individual or of society, but are of both.

One way in which values in healthcare have been described is as a 'programme' of spirituality and spiritual values (Eagger *et al.*, 2005). While this may not be mainstream to the values-based practice, it provides a useful alternative approach that offers a way of understanding spirituality as an adjunct to or substitute for secular values. Three principles underpin the scheme: physician heal thyself – that health care practitioners 'cannot aim to heal others before nurturing and healing themselves'; learning through experience, and being understood 'through direct "inner"' experience; and relevance to work

(Hewletta *et al.*, 2001) – seeking to manage exhausting work situations described as 'burnout' (Pines and Aronson, 2011). The values that are espoused are peace, positivity, compassion, cooperation, valuing the self and spirituality in healthcare. These have the advantage of evolving a provider mentality that is respectful, affirmative and empathetic, achieves reconciliation and is holistic and supportive. It is a philosophy of compassionate understanding that invades everyone and regulates the overall space within which thoughtful and kind actions occur. For a commissioner, it describes the outcome or objective of the system.

Using these values in practice will challenge commissioners to address and reflect on the way we deal with those who are exhausted, damaged, or in distress. We must ensure that the values of compassionate caring are made real. All healthcare situations reveal the need to make the caring process one that is supportive without paternalism and therapeutic without being repressive. If we consider the values pertaining to services, we note that most have values that are lenses through which we view ourselves and the world, the basis for our thoughts, feelings, and behaviour, and ideas by which we evaluate ourselves and others. Values tend to be standards we hold, which we experience as 'shoulds' and 'oughts', and are highly influential in the way we make decisions. Our values are satisfied when we take part in activities or that express those values. Conflict can occur if a person holds competing values that prevent him or her from participating fully in one valued role because of a clash of values with another area of her life.

Values motivate us to do certain things and not others, and are an important characteristic of who we are (Eagger *et al.*, 2005; Cornell University, 2011). For example, most people hold that addressing health inequalities, and acting to ensure there is no adverse discrimination, are values worth protecting. Cornell University, as just one example of many, offers a number of statements on diversity that demonstrate a positive dimension to their attitudes.

- Commitment to equitable treatment and elimination of discrimination in all its forms at all organisational levels.
- Commitment to diversity in all staff, volunteers and audiences, including full participation in programs, policy formulation, and decision-making.
- Recognition of the rights of all individuals to mutual respect.
- Acceptance of others without biases based on differences of any kind.
- Ability to lead and model diversity throughout the organisation and to lead society toward pluralism.
- Commitment to individual and organisational efforts to build respect, dignity, fairness, caring, equality, and self-esteem. (Cornell University, 2011)

The elements of a strong anti-discriminatory programme are centred on respect; and by themselves set the values face of the organisation firmly towards equality.

Conclusion

Values-based practice requires a strong commitment to engaging stakeholders in a variety of ways, as we shall see in more detail later, to understand the divergent values in the community and use those values to prepare a filter for the evidence. In Chapter 3 we will see the extent to which values and evidence form a new narrative rationality on which to make these critical decisions.

Chapter 2

Policy and practice

Values

Values are found in many places (Picture of Values, 2009). There are values inherent or expressed in relevant legislation and related policy positions; values determined by communities, groups and individuals; values developed or engaged for a variety of reasons, such as ethical systems or priority-setting schemes; and values inherent in a specific professional role or discipline or determined through training and education. Values do not have to be those that would underpin an ethical scheme. Those values may be concerned with equity, equality, beneficence, non-malfeasance, justice and autonomy. However, values may be much more prosaic, reflecting and dependent on real-life concerns, such as treating a person with dignity, respect, tolerance and understanding.

Values-based practice is a process that supports balanced decision-making within a framework of shared values where complex and conflicting values are in play (Fulford *et al.*, 2012, forthcoming). Values-based commissioning aims to support balanced decision-making within a framework of shared or negotiated values based on the 'premise of mutual respect and relying for its practical effectiveness on good process' rather than on previously arranged right answers. We may have a set of answers that we genuinely believe are the 'right' outcomes, but so may others. Negotiating values will enable us to respond respectfully to the wishes and demands of others in a way that preserves and indeed enhances our own values, even when we agree that the others' values will trump.

The Mental Health Act 2007, which amended the Act of 1983, has within Section 8 a set of principles (or values) that 'the Secretary of State thinks should inform decisions under this Act'. In preparing the statement of principles the Secretary of State shall, 'in particular, ensure' that each of a set of matters is addressed. These include:

(a) respect for patients' past and present wishes and feelings;
(b) respect for diversity generally, including, in particular, diversity of religion, culture and sexual orientation;
(c) minimising restrictions on liberty;
(d) involvement of patients in planning, developing and delivering care and treatment appropriate to them;
(e) avoidance of unlawful discrimination;
(f) effectiveness of treatment;
(g) views of carers and other interested parties;
(h) patient well-being and safety; and
(i) public safety.

Additionally, Section 8 says that 'the Secretary of State shall have regard to', inter alia, the:

(a) efficient use of resources; and

(b) equitable distribution of services.

These principles sum up what amounts to a distinct and substantial opportunity for values-based practice to develop and for patients, service users and carers to be given a much greater say in the planning, development and delivery of support care and treatment. If all the principles were to be enacted as they stand, it would change dramatically the nature and bureaucracy of care. Nonetheless, the principles do not overturn the purpose of legislation and leave out a number of high-profile aspects of care. For example, diversity of 'religion, culture and sexual orientation' does not include age, disability, gender or ethnicity. It might be thought that these would be considered under avoidance of unlawful discrimination, and indeed that is where particular matters may lodge.

However, a well-developed, values-based practice will insist that diversity must include all those matters covered by the Equalities Act 2010 with a set of values that support an Equalities Strategy. This includes age, ethnicity, gender, disability, faith and religion, carers, sexual orientation and economic status. An equality strategy is a vision for a strong, modern and fair community, built on two principles of equality – equal treatment and equal opportunity (Equalities Act, 2010). Implementing the Act such that discrimination does not exist will challenge many commissioners, especially the need under V-BP to include the views of patients, service users and carers.

The Mental Capacity Act 2005 sets out a series of principles that are not value-free. They include that a person must be assumed to have capacity unless it is established that he lacks capacity, and he is not to be treated as unable to make a decision unless all practicable steps to help him to do so have been taken without success. Additionally, a person is not to be treated as unable to make a decision merely because he makes an unwise decision (Mental Capacity Act 2005, Section 4). Our values come into play in determining when the person in question has capacity. There is a paradox: he is not to be treated as incapacitated until it is determined he lacks capacity, but it is not possible to determine whether he has capacity without undertaking some form of test. More interestingly is the question of what is an 'unwise' decision. This turns on our value judgements about what is unwise. Is looking after one cat? Or forty cats? Or 400 cats? It will depend on his circumstances. However, a simple assumption of incapacity is unacceptable.

Other sources of values include our upbringing, home life, school or college, religion or faith, whether we have disabilities, and so on. An example was provided by the Department of Health in 2005. When senior staff responsible for the minimum data set (MDS) associated with mental health care were asked why the data did not include information on religion, they appeared incredulous that anyone would want to know. It took quite a lot of effort to obtain agreement to include a question about religion in the national mental health census. The senior staff values were secular to the point of denying religion mattered, and they did not seem to accept or understand the importance of faith to many people.

Other systems of values that have been enshrined in legislation include the Health and Social Care Bill 2011 that proposes clinical commissioning groups and Health and Well-being Boards, with greater market opportunities for the private and third sectors. This value is significant. The present government's view is to want more competition and to offer the independent sector the chance to develop in competition with the NHS. (This is covered in more detail in Chapter 3.) The range of values is wide. For instance, the Data Protection Act has a number of values that might at first sight seem less appropriate although they are mandatory and good practice. These include eight principles:

- fairly and lawfully processed;
- processed for limited purposes;
- adequate, relevant and not excessive;
- accurate and up-to-date;
- not kept for longer than is necessary;
- processed in line with your rights;
- secure; and
- not transferred to other countries without adequate protection.

These eight principles then give rise to a set of rights including safeguarding, accessing and correcting information, preventing the processing of information, unsolicited marketing and automated decision-making, and claiming compensation. Similarly, the Freedom of Information Act gives a person the right to request official information held by public authorities, unless there are good reasons to keep it confidential. However, this does not go far enough for some. For example, the Human Rights Organisation, Article 19, has set out nine areas of the Freedom of Information Act (FOIA) that it suggests should be strengthened, including maximum disclosure and an obligation to publish, with limited scope for exceptions, promotion of open government and processes to facilitate access, disclosure taking precedence over non-disclosure, and protection for whistle-blowers. These values would require a much more open government process.

Again, the principles that inform the government's approach to EU legislation include the statement that, '[W]herever possible, the Government will argue for alternatives to regulation at European level' (Guiding Principles for EU legislation, 2011, accessed 21 July 2011). Although not concerned directly with health and social care, the statement proposes that wherever possible regulation will be done on the basis of subsidiarity – i.e. at the lowest level that it is effective. This finds useful expression in health and social care, which is by and large provided locally. Another area where values are mostly commercial but which establish parameters for other areas is in the process of procurement for *sustainable* development. Some would argue that this is generally unnecessary these days as many people have become committed to sustainable practice. Unfortunately, there is more in the belief than in the deed. Nonetheless, procurement is an aspect of service development that we cannot ignore, and doing so with a mind towards sustainability is a value that is held to a greater or lesser extent.

Following the Bruntland Report 1997, sustainability has become an essential requirement for 'development which meets the needs of the present without compromising the ability of future generations to meet their own needs'. As with other aspects of commissioning, this is a factor that some, more than others, may consider important. For example, commissioning services from a hospital may require a carbon footprint to be described and acted upon. In its way this will not affect patients directly or immediately, but it might impact on patients when they see it used, for example, as a reason or excuse to increase car parking charges. Climate change, which we will touch on briefly in Chapter 7, suggests a further set of values, both about the role of everyone in seeking to limit global warming, but especially the role of public health in tackling the health-related consequences.

The NHS Constitution is another place where an agreed set of 'community' values has been enshrined in a way that is often more remarked upon in the word than the deed. (The Constitution is reproduced in the Annex to this chapter.) The seven areas of the Constitution include access to services, the quality of care and the environment, informed choice and the right to information. Within each of the seven areas, patients have positive rights *to* certain goods such as maximum waiting times or drug treatments recommended by a doctor, but even these values are open to careful questioning. For example, to what extent is information to be made available? To what extent is there an opportunity 'to be involved directly or through representatives, in the planning of healthcare services, the development and consideration of proposals for changes in the way those services are provided, and in decisions to be made affecting the operation of those services' (NHS Constitution)? This is critical if V-BP is to achieve the necessary changes sought. As we saw earlier, the use of representative bodies is one important strand of planning services. Using a 'thick' rather than the too-often used 'thin' mechanism (see below), means doing exactly what the Constitution says: involvement in planning health care, changing (commissioning) the service, and operation of the NHS systems.

Values-based practice is the other side of the coin of evidence-based practice; the two go together. Evidence is read through values, not alone. However, often the idea of values arises tangentially as evidence becomes weak or is non-existent. And values are logically prior to evidence. The evidence relevant to health and social care is large and increasingly unwieldy, but still the evidence can be made more intelligible by filtering it through a values-based net. We may not know everything about the values espoused by a particular group, but we can consider what the critical aspects of a service might be and ask some searching questions before we even set the evidence a real values-based test.

Balancing guidelines with values and innovation

One way of looking at it is from a 'full field' perspective – this philosophical approach seeks to understand the nature of responses in mental disorder. One half-field is concerned with function, the other half with action. Facts (disease) cash out as a failure of function; values (illness) cash out as failure of action. So the first approach is to say that if we have only the E-BP element we will not realise all the benefits of ascertaining values and be concerned only with function and not with the wider agency of the person(s) with mental health problems.

A second approach is to see values as offering a way to understand the evidence. By focusing on values we are able to filter the evidence through them and this determines the use of the evidence that is available. In the case of NICE, where it offers a range of options (which it does not in all cases) we can use values-based commissioning to understand and relate the evidence to values. NICE guidance is predicated on different types of scientific evidence. The gold standard is the meta-analysis of randomised controlled trials (RCTs), but there is a range of methodological rigour from which it draws. Its advantage is the ability for everyone to know what is going on: replicability of interventions and a clear relationship with professionalism. This means that we know the credentials of people able to administer the interventions, the length of a course of treatment, how much it costs, and so forth. Its disadvantages are the limitations of research methodology (application to real life, inequity in enrolment, effect size, etc.); exclusion of interventions that do not lend themselves to application-hungry or time-constrained researchers (e.g. psychodynamic psychotherapy); and an over-reliance on evidence-based medicine by medical (and medicalised) services. This is unsurprising given the emphasis on E-BP during the 'noughties', but that is why V-BP is so important: to redress the balance and ensure that values and people are brought back fully and explicitly into the fold.

When NICE is unsure then it is easier to offer alternatives. However, this becomes more problematic where NICE (or any other national agency) suggests only one offer, and that offer is challenged by the values of some (or indeed all) members of a group or community. Here we need to recognise that there will be two related strategies: (1) to encourage innovation and/or research and to try new treatments or service responses possibly on an experimental basis –if successful, these then become additions to the treatment modalities available; and (2) to address the problem using a resource allocation methodology – Programme Budgeting and Marginal Analysis (PBMA) with a range of cost–quality indicators, linked of course to deontological elements (see Chapter 8 on priority setting). In other words, any effective resource allocation must balance cost–benefit or cost–utility systems with rights to treatment especially (although not exclusively) where there is prior discrimination.

Cost–benefit calculations will not always address health inequalities, but a rights-based approach will not address arguments about fairness. It is here that we may want to look at allocative efficiency as one option – this will work if there is sufficient information, but will not be adequate if there are differing levels or types of information available. While health provides evidence-based medicine, local government coordinates or, in some cases, provides social interventions. Values-based commissioning enables equity of esteem between the 'facts' of evidence-based medicine and social care, and the 'values' of values-based medicine and social care. Thus, allocative efficiency is a shared objective between health and social care with each respecting the traditions and relevance of the other.

Finally, some forms of treatment, care or support are so different and distinct that they will need to be tried by the service users separately or at least by service users with some support. This is a challenge to those who espouse service user leadership and management of services. Will we allow service users to decide that the services on offer are simply not appropriate and that they should be allowed to devise their own (from a values-based perspective) to use? There will need to be a system for deciding who might be allowed to do this, when and on what criteria. In part, this is about a proper recognition of minority concerns and suggests a political rather than simply a bureaucratic response. It does, after all, beg the question of whether NICE is always right; and in turn this raises a further question as to whether the values of the users (or anyone else for that matter) are always right!

National Guidelines actively encourage taking into account individuals' needs and preferences; support the involvement of patients and carers in decision-making; and suggest that psychosocial interventions of the sort that might be more attractive to patients than drugs and cognitive-behavioural therapy (CBT). There is thus some room for manoeuvre. The state (the NHS and local authorities) has to have a peg on which to hang the guidance it gives. What should be offered as a statutory service, free at the point of delivery? Evidence-based medicine provides one set of information about which (if it is based on good research) there can be little argument. Values-based practice opens up an altogether different set of arguments.

The potential power of the concepts of 'right care' and 'value' appear when an innovation or an idea becomes sufficiently evaluated to enable dissemination through commissioning. Thus, the establishment of quality improvement or productivity of a service development becomes another manifestation of 'evidence' on which decisions about expending public money can be made.

Does an approach that spends most of the 'health' money on evidence-based medicine, and most of the local authority money on picking up the pieces of failed prevention, constitute the right advice? No. Health and social care resources need to be pooled and aimed in the first instance at cost–benefit-proven universal and targeted individual and population interventions. Values-based practice may offer some practical solutions. Let us take the example of a group of patients that state what they want is a, b and c, and these are cheaper than evidence-based medicine. There may an ethical argument to invest in a, b and c at the expense of E-BP because: (1) it supports funding of prevention/wellness services; (2) it makes illness services more affordable and therefore more available; and (3) a, b and c are what patients want anyway. However, what happens if one or more of a, b, and c are not only *not* well-evidenced but positively harmful. Is there an ethical argument in their favour? To resolve the dilemma demands full engagement with patients and service users.

'Thin' and 'thick' systems

At this point it is important to describe what may be called the 'weak' or 'thin' and the 'strong' or 'thick' notions of V-BP. Because much of values-based discourse is based on 'involvement' rather than 'participation', it leads to a weaker version of V-BP that we might refer to as 'thin'. 'Thin' suggests a rather different interpretation to 'weak' – it is as robust, but does not contain all the components that we might need for a fully rounded approach. In the thin version, patients, service users and carers have the right to be involved, to be approached, consulted and listened to, and to have their ideas and thoughts considered in the development of treatment care and support. Involvement can take a number of forms (see Chapter 5), but at root it is a limited exercise that listens respectfully but where the professional commissioner remains the final arbiter to make whatever decisions are required. They (patients and service users) are not and do not become commissioners.

The 'strong' or 'thick' notion of V-BP takes the process much further, and offers all those engaged the opportunity to negotiate values, to review the evidence as equal partners, and to participate fully with commissioners, as commissioners, in the debates and decisions about the development of care. In this 'thick' option, 'commissioners' become all those who have an interest (within reasonable bounds) in making decisions about care support and treatment.

Table 2.1 'Thin' and 'thick' systems for values-based practice.

	Individual	Group	Community	Population
'Thin' systems	Require a simple approach that recognises certain basic features	Requires that one or more groups have developed a set of values	Simple community values that are engaged on a generic basis	A generic approach accepting national guidelines
'Thick' systems	Require a full assessment and recognition of the values of the individual	Demand a system to recognise the values of the relevant groups involved (by age, gender, faith, etc.) Require a compromise between individual and group values	Complex community values demanding a detailed approach to *all* relevant (and diverse) groups in the community	A complex multi-faceted system for drawing out information democratically and ensuring implementation

We can see this in the following example from mental health services. The mental health service commissioners, GPs and other professional staff have agreed to develop a service user advisory group to offer advice and guidance to commissioners. One of the GPs has agreed to undertake an evaluation of the process. This suggested that the group has some valuable ideas and recommends a number of improvements in the structure, representation and process of the group. However, the group is still largely tokenist, and thus to some extent marginalised. Although it has become *involved* it does not have the *participatory* flavour of the thick system. By and large, patients and service users have little experience of such groups and are pleased that it exists, is listened to and its views acted on to a degree. The membership is fluid, made up for the time being of those who are well and have an interest. The commissioners argue that it can be nothing more demanding as they have a job to do and cannot be held up by a process that engages more patients, service users or carers.

Is this adequate? The thick version does go much further. In this there is process of transformation based on a participatory process with a network arrangement that is more robust. Two factors make this possible: first, recognition that there are many views and values which have not been tapped into, or taken into account; and second, that there are many people who do not want to be involved all the time but whose values should be considered regularly and taken into account in negotiation. The sort of network which will work is one normally based on the operation of biological neural systems; however, for our purposes we are concerned only with what is important about such networks. It is essentially a parallel processing system.

The advantages of parallel systems are that they can perform tasks that a linear process cannot, especially because if an element of the network fails, the rest of the network can continue without a problem by virtue of its parallel nature. Neural networks learn and do not need to be reprogrammed. There are, however, some disadvantages: a neural network needs 'training' to operate effectively (but that would be needed in any event); and the architecture is different from that of the usual systems of involvement and thus needs to be developed and supported.

What does a parallel network look like in practice? Instead of a linear system, a neural network is a parallel system that includes a range of people that can form the 'aura' or 'halo' of information.

The traditional approach has an element of bureaucracy that limits the way in which the main group can develop, change or evolve. This would be a star or simple arrangement in which the outlying groups are included by some representative mechanism. Conversely, a parallel network offers the opportunity to have a range of people, some patients or service users, some carers, some people from professional groups, participating in the determination of care options (see Figure 2.1). Each of these can be more or less autonomous as long as there is a mechanism to bring the groups' deliberations together. Simple systems suffer from the problem of sustainability; parallel networks offer longer-term engagement with opportunities for all stakeholders to be involved.

One concern that has been expressed is that this is (or at least may become) time-consuming, when commissioners have a lot to do in a short time and need to 'get on with it'. In practice, as we can see here, this form of network offers the option of regular updates on values, a process of consultation, and a way that many more patients/service users, and carers, can be engaged. Neural networks learn from the questions asked and change their nature and response depending on the answers. Similarly, the systems that commissioners need to develop will have forms of built-in-learning that ensure the process does not

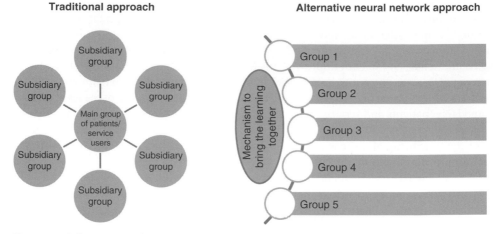

Figure 2.1 Differing approaches to service user and staff engagement.

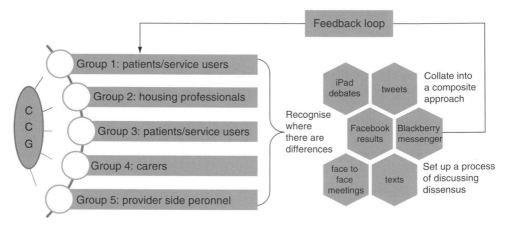

Figure 2.2 A mechanism for engaging service users with digital technology.

continually ask the same questions, but accepts the thrust of patients and service-user values and focuses on those values that differ and require negotiation.

More importantly, the use of new technology and digital systems offer ways to tap into the values of patients, service users, professionals and the public. Digital systems (mobile phones, Twitter, Facebook, and so on) provide many ways in which commissioners can regularly, and if necessary frequently, ask sections of the population or specialist groups about their values and the way those values might impact on commissioner decisions. Twitter is used increasingly by politicians and celebrities, institutions with messages to impart such as universities, businesses that want to bring their message to a wide range of people, and ordinary folk with a view on the world. You can sign up to the tweets of an individual, or get all the tweets from a journal, art gallery or pension service. The scope is more or less unlimited (as shown in Figure 2.2).

Facebook is a social networking site used by many younger people and increasingly by sections of the whole population. By establishing a Facebook site with critical questions on a

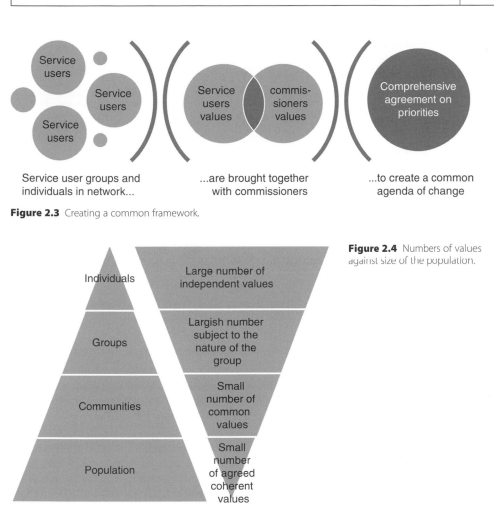

Figure 2.3 Creating a common framework.

Service user groups and individuals in network...

...are brought together with commissioners

...to create a common agenda of change

Figure 2.4 Numbers of values against size of the population.

subject, it may be possible to engage an ever-widening group of people with similar interests. Text and text messengers, use of iPads and similar tablet computers as well as face-to-face meetings all allow values to be obtained and analysed without extensive and time-consuming work.

Such a network gives commissioners the chance to talk to a range of stakeholders regularly, to negotiate values, and to develop proposals for change that have been considered by a wide range of patients and professional staff. Of course, no mechanism takes away responsibility from the commissioner to work closely with service users or other professional staff. Indeed, commissioners need to work with service-users-as-commissioners in addition to the mechanisms suggested above. (See Figure 2.3.)

Developing this system suggests that a distinction must be made between the individual and the population perspective, or indeed three different population approaches: the group of people with similar characteristics; a 'community', which will probably be geographical but may be faith-based, age-related, or clustered on another common factor; and the wider national or regional population. By considering the interplay of the thick and thin systems we can see the nature of the demands that values-based commissioning places on commissioners, as shown in Figure 2.4 and Table 2.1.

Table 2.2 Population and individual factors.

	Risk profiles	Personalised services	Shared decisions
Population	Public health, epidemiological information, and clinical knowledge	Policy based on population values about personalised services	Programme of information to patients/service users
Individual	Risk-based discussion with the individual patient about personal circumstances	Individual care plan based on a values discussion	Discussion with individual patients on needs, wishes and values

Long-term care provides an interesting example. Around 15 million people live with a long-term condition in England, and they account for roughly 70% of overall health and care spend (QIPP Workstreams, 2011). Consequently, any improvement in their use of the NHS and social care, and thus improvements in clinical outcomes and experience, will have a disproportionately positive effect. The QIPP programme focuses on improving the quality and productivity of services so that patients and service users and their carers can access higher-quality, local, comprehensive community and primary care. Three principles underpin the work.

- Risk profiles, to enable commissioners to manage those at risk and to agree targets and priorities.
- Neighbourhood care teams, to provide joined up and personalised services in the community.
- Self-care and shared decision-making, including a 'systematic transfer of knowledge and power' to patients and service users, with the co-production of a care plan.

Each of these is important of itself for values-based commissioning, and together they form an important set of features of the process. Risk profiling provides both a population and an individual risk profile enabling services to be offered that are tailored to the needs, wishes and values of the patient or service user. Personalised services allow that to happen effectively; the self-care and shared decision-making makes explicit the claim of 'no decision about me without me'; and patients become active participants in deciding their care.

From a values-based *commissioning* perspective, these features suggest at least a two-level programme: the population level and the individual level. By developing a programme of values-based discussion with the patient(s) or service user(s), it will be possible to understand the way in which the values of the patient(s) can be accommodated as shown in Table 2.2.

Conclusion

Values-based practice can be undertaken fully (thick systems) or at a much reduced level (thin systems). It will be evident that the thin approach is not sufficient for a substantial values understanding. The thin system is the minimum necessary to be able to say, 'we have listened to the values of service users'. However, to 'hear' those values demands a much more comprehensive and inclusive approach in which commissioners engage patients and service users regularly and completely. By doing so, the exercise becomes fulfilling and rewarding, and the health and social care that results will be much more acceptable to those who use the services.

Annex 1

NHS Constitution

Access to health services: the right to:

- receive NHS services free of charge;
- access NHS services;
- expect your local NHS to assess the health requirements of the local community and to commission and put in place the services to meet those needs as considered necessary;
- not be unlawfully discriminated against in the provision of NHS services including on grounds of gender, race, religion or belief, sexual orientation, disability (including learning disability or mental illness) or age;
- access services within maximum waiting times, or for the NHS to take all reasonable steps to offer you a range of alternative providers if this is not possible.

Quality of care and environment: the right to:

- be treated with a professional standard of care, by appropriately qualified and experienced staff, in a properly approved or registered organisation that meets required levels of safety and quality;
- expect NHS organisations to monitor, and make efforts to improve, the quality of healthcare they commission or provide.

Nationally approved treatments, drugs and programmes: the right to:

- drugs and treatments that have been recommended by NICE for use in the NHS, if recommended by your doctor;
- expect local decisions on funding of other drugs and treatments to be made rationally following a proper consideration of the evidence;
- receive the vaccinations that the Joint Committee on Vaccination and Immunisation recommends that you should receive under an NHS-provided national immunisation programme.

Respect, consent and confidentiality: the right to:

- be treated with dignity and respect, in accordance with your human rights;
- accept or refuse treatment that is offered to you, and not to be given any physical examination or treatment unless you have given valid consent;
- be given information about your proposed treatment in advance, including any significant risks and any alternative treatments which may be available, and the risks involved in doing nothing;
- privacy and confidentiality and to expect the NHS to keep your confidential information safe and secure;
- access to your own health records which will always be used to manage your treatment in your best interests.

Informed choice: the right to:

- choose your GP practice, and to be accepted by that practice unless there are reasonable grounds to refuse, and you will be informed of those reasons;
- express a preference for using a particular doctor within your GP practice, and for the practice to try to comply;
- make choices about your NHS care and to information to support these choices.

Involvement in your healthcare and in the NHS: the right to:

- be involved in discussions and decisions about your healthcare, and to be given information to enable you to do this;
- be involved directly or through representatives, in the planning of healthcare services, the development and consideration of proposals for changes in the way those services are provided, and in decisions to be made affecting the operation of those services.

Complaint and redress: the right to:

- have any complaint you make about NHS services dealt with efficiently and to have it properly investigated;
- know the outcome of any investigation into your complaint;
- take your complaint to the independent Health Service Ombudsman, if you are not satisfied with the way your complaint has been dealt with by the NHS;
- make a claim for judicial review if you think you have been directly affected by an unlawful act or decision of an NHS body;
- compensation where you have been harmed by negligent treatment.

'The NHS also commits:

- to inform you about the healthcare services available to you, locally and nationally;
- to provide you with the information you need to influence and scrutinise the planning and delivery of NHS services;
- to offer you easily accessible, reliable and relevant information to enable you to participate fully in your own healthcare decisions and to support you in making choices. This will include information on the quality of clinical services where there is robust and accurate information available;
- to work in partnership with you, your family, carers and representatives.'

Chapter 3

Health and social care reforms in England

The health and social care reforms in England are an opportunity to develop an innovative programme that marries values and evidence and that is at once person-centred and clinically sound. Values-based practice is not dependent on the reforms: if the reforms did not occur, this would still be the right time to establish more effective processes of clinical commissioning; but conversely given that the reforms may occur, then the opportunity should be taken to improve the values basis of decision-making. Many burgeoning strands of action demonstrate this: the QIPP 'Right Care' programme (2011), an emphasis on shared decision-making, attempts to achieve integration, and a focus on GP-led clinical commissioning, all point to a gathering of opinion that will become an unstoppable force for change. Engaging GPs and other clinicians in an integrative process that encourages values-based and evidence-based practice as a shared approach to improving the doctor–patient and professional–service user relationships in the context of a population perspective.

Primary care commissioning: historical precedents

Previous attempts at ensuring that evidence and local values were in harmony have had a mixed press. Since the advent of the internal market in 1991, a number of initiatives have been tried to get primary care physicians more engaged in commissioning. From fund-holding during the early 90s to practice-based commissioning, there has been a succession of mechanisms proposed, each of which has been found wanting by one section of society or another.

Following the NHS and Community Care Act 1990, the NHS was divided into purchasers (predominantly, at the outset, health authorities) and providers (NHS Trusts). Over a period of four or five years, all providers moved from being directly managed units (DMUs) to being autonomous trusts within the NHS; and health authorities, via a series of mergers and developments, established fund-holding arrangements for general practice. Fund-holding practices received budgets to cover three elements of their responsibilities: ancillary practice staff, a range of non-emergency hospital (elective) services, and prescribing (Keeley, 1997; Kings Fund, 2010). Savings made on these budgets could be used to support other areas, or be spent in other ways to enhance services to patients. These 'real' budgets were intended as an incentive to GP practices to manage cost and apply some competitive pressure on providers (Kings Fund, 2010). Some GP practices worked together in consortia and in 1994 a total purchasing scheme was introduced that encouraged GP practices (either singly or in groups) to take the whole budget on an indicative basis to commission all services.

Fund-holding had mixed success, but the main factor that led to its demise was the claim that it had created a two-tier health service: patients in fund-holding practices were considered to have better access to health care than those in non-fund-holding practices

(Kay, 2002). This analysis did not give much credence either to the (relatively minor) improvements made by fund-holding (and total purchasing pilots (TPPs) particularly), or to the values and evidence debate. Fund-holding is a highly value-laden enterprise, and places a premium on local decision-making and local accountability. Within these we can make explicit the trust that was expected in the GP as clinical commissioner, and a recognition of improvements bought by the fund-holder. The other side of this coin was the charge of two tier services, high transaction costs, a post code lottery in prescribing especially (Le Grand *et al.*, 1998). Fund-holding GPs appear to have achieved quicker admissions for their patients and shorter waiting times (Dowling, 2000).

As important was the allegation that some doctors had (entirely legally) transferred capital purchases to personal assets on the balance sheet. By making savings on health care budgets, GPs were able to fund new and sometimes quite palatial surgeries, which they themselves owned. Was this an example of early adopters setting and achieving higher standards, or was it blatant profiteering? This raised other questions. Should doctors (or indeed other health care practitioners) make money from patients (other than in the form of salary)? What level of differentiation is acceptable between different parts of the NHS, especially when there is a level of innovation, which may in the end benefit everyone? How can changes be made sustainable rather than short-lived opportunities which by their nature will need to be ended quite quickly (such as the transfer of assets)? This goes to the heart of our values within the NHS, and also more widely within society. The question about doctors' remuneration, for example, would not spur the same concern in the USA, where many doctors are based in private practice and would expect to be able to maximise their income (possibly within some overall regulated ceiling). Economic and cultural values come into contention. In the USA (at the time of writing) health care costs had risen to more than 17% of GDP with 45 million Americans uninsured.

Total purchasing pilots were of variable quality and their experience was small scale and highly localised (Mays *et al.*, 2001). Some, however, challenged provider hospital procedures, especially, on the one hand, the 'gaming' that had developed where some hospitals would make sequential consultant-to-consultant referrals without recourse to the GP, and on the other, seeking to bring health and social care together in dealing, for example, with teenage pregnancy or appropriate accommodation on discharge of mentally ill people from hospital. Transaction costs were higher, though, largely as a result of establishing appropriate management and consultation procedures. Following the abolition of fund-holding by the Labour government in 1997, health authorities created primary care groups, and in time these merged and migrated to become primary care trusts (PCTs), with the abolition of the parent health authorities; and at the same time Strategic Health Authorities were borne.

In 2004, the government announced the creation of practice-based commissioning (PbC). PbC was not compulsory: practices could choose to participate (in various configurations) and be given an indicative budget along with data on the volume and cost of services, such as in-patient elective care, or A&E attendances. Practices were then allowed to make savings to reinvest in existing or new services (Kings Fund, 2010). PbC was not generally successful or welcomed, although it provided a test bed in some areas that enabled GPs to experiment with funding options (Curry *et al.*, 2010). GPs have not been able to engage effectively with PbC consortia, and many do not have the necessary commissioning skills (Wood and Curry, 2009). A lack of incentives, disagreements on objectives and a 'cumbersome PCT bureaucracy' (Kings Fund, 2010).

Overall, the evidence for effective primary care-led commissioning is slight. Implementation barriers have had an impact, such as effective local organisational arrangements and negotiation with providers, plus constant reorganisations; obtaining a commitment to engage with clinical commissioning; and values-based disparities between practices on the desirability of practice-based processes. As we move forward with Clinical Commissioning Groups (CCGs), we need to ask a number of (often values-based) questions: what objectives will clinical commissioners set, how will they be agreed, and who will agree them? Will CCGs have sufficient resources for a reasonable and sensitive engagement with the local population? If so, how will patients and service users be engaged? Will GPs be expected to lead and 'do' commissioning, or will they have management staff do it for them under their direction? (Supporting evidence-based decisions, 2011.)

As CCGs develop they will inevitably require a lot of support and assistance, much of which may come from commercial organisations whose values may differ sharply from those of the NHS (Light, 2011). However, as the values of primary care change (for example, GPs are less willing to take on out-of-hours provision), commercialisation of support may be more attractive as long as it does not leave patients to fend for themselves. Many patients want care protocols that are more expensive than the state wishes to provide. For example, patients want to be cared for at home, but beyond some levels of basic care, to do so is expensive. Will we see patients' values ignored in the drive for cost improvement, savings and efficiency, or will we see a better balance of economy and effectiveness that trades on a careful discussion of values and evidence to achieve a solution acceptable to the patient and agreeable to the commissioner (Sell, 2010)?

Values-base of the government's reforms

Let us begin this section by considering the values base of the reforms, even though some of what is discussed may seem to be of historical interest only. Unfortunately, the reforms were sold to an unsuspecting public as a 'necessity'. It was argued that the NHS needed reform and the proposals in the White Paper Equity and Excellence: Liberating the NHS (Department of Health, 2010) were offered as an essential change, one that could not be shirked. Many people in England accepted the challenge initially, including a large number of family doctors, some of whom were encouraged by the chance to take greater responsibility for commissioning. Initially the proposals went down fairly well and did not at that stage cause the stir marked by the government's unprecedented 'pause' on the legislation. To some degree this was achieved by the Deputy Prime Minister when he spoke about his concerns about the Bill (see, for example, the blog at http://www.guardian.co.uk/society/blog/2011/may/26/nhs-reforms-live-blog). Until that time, he and other Liberal Democrats had supported the general stance of the Bill and were in accord with the main planks of policy contained within it.

By and large, the original White Paper ideas had been accepted for three reasons. First, the NHS does as it's told, especially if it likes what it sees. That may not have been the case here, but there were sufficient incentives for NHS managers to support the changes – at least initially. Any major change is a headache, but the NHS knuckles down and makes the changes usually sooner than (or at least as quickly as) the politicians expect. David Cameron (Prime Minister) and Andrew Lansley (Secretary of State for Health) were surprised; David Nicholson (NHS Chief Executive) was not. Second, the proposals made some sort of sense. If we are to change the way services are commissioned, preferably for the better, then the loss of PCTs and the opportunity to give resources to GPs and colleagues seemed like a good idea. PCTs had not covered themselves in glory, although maybe they were just beginning to take the necessary decisions and to make inroads into commissioning decisions. Local government, by the same token, had realised that social care commissioning required a closer relationship with health. GPs noted that the policy contained a conflict of interest (between commissioning and providing as GP practices), but that could be put to one side in the greater good of the NHS and social care, and of course for a small number, the opportunity to privatise parts or all of it.

Third, the NHS commissioning arms reacted with great speed to the overall position with which it was confronted. With commissioning described even by its supporters as slow and cumbersome (Kings Fund, 2010), and with opportunities for early retirement, it was no surprise that staff who could took their pensions (or locked in the opportunity to do so within two years). This meant that PCTs that were expected to keep commissioning going for two or three years had, by spring 2011, more or less lost the will to commission effectively, or had become unable to function. Some staff had gone back to Strategic Health Authorities (SHAs) to pick up the challenge of commissioning through GP consortia, and to encourage behaviour changes among GPCC (GP Commissioning Consortia); some staff had joined acute or mental health trusts; the rest had retired or been made redundant, either immediately or in a short space of time.

What does this tell us about the underlying values of the NHS and local authorities? First, that there is far too much opportunism (and some lack of principle) within the health service especially; and second, that the NHS as a national body will do more or less what it is told, slavishly some might say, with little murmur. Albeit that this is not a pretty trait, it has served the NHS well over the years. In this case, of course, the government is intent on privatising, or causing to be privatised, large sections of the NHS, in addition to many local government services already privatised (and of the reminder the Localism Act will do the same job). The initial reaction by GPs to the GPCC proposals was, at one end of the spectrum, one of genuine interest among a small section of those who want greater freedoms to manage their own affairs; at the other end, outright greed among a small number of businessmen-GPs intent on using the reforms to fashion privatised vehicles for personal profit; and, in the middle, a large cohort of GPs who were either disinclined to get involved or who would do so when the fog of legislative war lifted.

Public values have been little tested. It is evident that there is a lot of love for the NHS although perhaps somewhat less for local government. However, by the way that the reforms have developed one would be forgiven for assuming that few people would mind if the NHS was broken up and privatised, but this is almost certainly incorrect. It takes time for the 'penny to drop'. Because of the government's approach there has been time for people 'to get their act together', almost literally, in that by late October 2011 peers had tabled over 300 amendments to the Act in the House of Lords, identifying a ground swell of opinion directed against the government's position. Values such as: support for a social contract or 'compact' including inter-generational cooperation; services that are comprehensive and funded out of general taxation, free at the point of use; maximum integration between health and social care; and state guarantees from cradle to grave care.

All these demonstrate that the population wants a health and social care service that is not only free at the point of delivery and funded out of general taxation, but managed by the state and governed in the best interests of the people. The NHS and social care support constitutes a commonwealth that is not amenable to privatisation. Private companies have a part to play, largely at the margins of mainstream care. The example of Southern Cross, a very large private nursing home provider that went into liquidation after the management team had taken excessive profits, entirely legally, shows what can happen if care is not legally sustainable, and financially sound within a carefully regulated environment.

The implications of these values were not lost on the government, however. The Liberal Democrats sought to paint the Coalition government as confused and out of touch; the Conservatives were so flummoxed that they insisted on stopping the Act and setting up a 'listening exercise'. In practice, this was unnecessary. If the government had simply pressed ahead they would have secured the changes that they wanted: a revised commissioning framework with GP commissioning groups, a contestable set of providers, revised public health, and local government taking control via Health and Well-being Boards. By pandering to the opposition both inside the Coalition, and within and outside Westminster, they have left themselves open to the charge of U-turns, lacking an understanding of the nature of their own reforms, and patently uncertain if the reforms will work. Yet it is evident, paradoxically, that the reforms could have been accepted if the proposals had been forced through. What doctors were saying in October 2010 was very different to what they said in June 2011 and different again from their position in early 2012.

This is not to argue that the reforms are either needed or helpful. It is simple realism, but not the whole story. The government has been both cautious and clever. Changes to the timetable for the end of PCTs have not changed, 'any qualified provider' is still an option, and GPs will become the main stay of the commissioning arrangements. Health and Well-being Boards were in any event unspecified and the changes suggest simply more of the story than had been told up to June 2011; many of the other 180-odd changes suggested after the 'pause' or 'listening exercise' will become the basis of a substantial amendment to the Bill. Monitor's role is the only casualty, but even then it will eventually be brought into contention. So the government has learned that the NHS has to appear to be safe even if it is not. The opposition's record on the changes was woeful. The details of the changes may seem unnecessary, but in the short term give away the government's intentions. Population values have been carefully manipulated to give the impression of status quo ante when the result is anything but!

Further changes

CCGs, a new designation that has replaced GPCC, will continue as groups of GP practices with an assurance that commissioning will involve patients, carers and the public and a wide range of doctors, nurses and other health and care professionals. They will have a duty to promote integrated health and social care to meet the needs of users, commission all urgent and emergency care, and take responsibility for unregistered patients in their area. No delegation of commissioning functions will be allowed to private companies or contractors, although whether social enterprises will be eligible is still uncertain. Each CCG will have 'at least two' lay members and two additional secondary care specialists, one a doctor and the other a nurse, drawn from a distant provider where no conflict exists; whether this will service implementation of the Bill (once passed) is unlikely.

If a CCG commissions effectively it may be eligible for a 'quality premium' which will be paid on the basis of rules still to be established (at October 2011) and which take into account the use of resources and evidence of outcomes. These unwritten rules allow extensive scope to the government to ride roughshod over opposition to the change. One of the constant refrains from GPs is the way that their relationship with patients and service users may be compromised; yet this was not, as a general rule, their first concern. Perhaps we will see a further about-turn if and when it becomes apparent that the new system is working and GPs can take direct responsibility for the budget. However, the government's intention to retain and strengthen cancer networks and other clinical areas, together with 'clinical senates' to give expert advice and to have a formal role in the authorisation of local CCGs, both complicates and attenuates the CCGs role.

Clinical senates, hosted directly by the NHS Commissioning Board, will give expert advice, ensure patient care fits together seamlessly, supports integration of care, and will include public health and adult and child social care experts. They will advise the NHS Commissioning Board on whether commissioning plans are clinically robust and on major changes. The outcome is thus a more complex bureaucratic system than at present and will, despite the stated intentions of the government, make change more difficult, not less. This is at a time when all commentators on the NHS believe that it requires at least a 10% reduction, if not more, in the number of hospitals and a significant shake up in the way patient care is managed. From a values-based commissioning perspective this situation is redolent of the past; the values of clinicians will take over from the values of the community or individuals.

Of all the alterations to the Act, the changes to Monitor's role are the most explicit. First, it will have to obtain appropriate clinical advice, although what that means is left rather vague. Second, Monitor's core role will be to protect and promote patients' interests. Third, Monitor's powers to 'promote' competition will be removed 'as if it were an end in itself'. What this means is unclear. Monitor will be limited to tackling specific abuses and unjustifiable restrictions that 'demonstrably act against patients' interests' so as to ensure a level playing field between providers. Monitor will be required to support the delivery of integrated services for patients where this would improve the quality of care for patients or improve efficiency.

In short, Monitor's role remains ambiguous. It may be seriously curtailed by the NHS Commissioning Board which will establish, in consultation with Monitor, the way that choice, competition, service bundling and integration will be effected. Monitor's powers over anti-competitive purchasing will focus on preventing abuses rather than competition, and its remit to open up competition will be removed. The Cooperation and Competition Panel (CCP) will become part of Monitor, alongside the concurrent powers (with the Office for Fair Trading, OFT) to ensure that competition rules can be applied by a sector-specific regulator with expertise in healthcare. Given that the EU competition panel rules will not change, the likely effect is to strengthen the competition arrangements rather than weaken them.

What is apparent about these changes and alterations is that the values of the community have had little impact. Most groups in the community want their local services to continue to develop effectively for them, and many did not want a lot of the changes that have been suggested. On the other hand, the idea of GPCC has found an acceptance; having GPs take responsibility may not have been appreciated by some, but for many others this was a change that seemed needed. PCTs had tried hard but unsuccessfully to develop good, accepted commissioning arrangements, although their success was just becoming visible when the rug was pulled from under their feet. There is therefore an opportunity now to reinstate values, to recognise the need to retrace our steps and as the changes take place put in place values-based commissioning.

Conclusion

The policy context does not demand values-based practice, but is a useful opportunity to insist on the 'value of values'. Whatever arrangement eventually emerges, values-based practice will be a necessary component. First, V-BC demands engagement of the community; and while CCGs may think they have a lot of more pressing priorities, working with patients and service users will inoculate CCGs and Health and Well-being Boards from the charge of top-down imposition of cuts. Second, in order to save £20 billion or more for reinvestment in health and social care, it will be essential to understand what patients and service users want and will put up with.

Evidence and outcomes: commissioning for value

4

Seven fat years: seven lean years

Commissioning health and social care services is both a cyclical programme and a progressive and extended process over a period of years. The idea of the commissioning cycle has been promoted by central government, but in reality most commissioners have neither the time nor the inclination to rewrite commissioner intentions, develop tender proposals or re-apply national contracts (assuming that is necessary every three years). As national contracts have become the norm with payment by results (PbR) the nature of the cycle has changed and now reflects an extended timeframe. The acceptance of a delaying structure is curious when the government is keen to extend market-based ideology into the health (and to a lesser extent social care) services.

The financial position of any commissioner is critical to the development of care. Contract management of agreements, possibly with ceilings and floors, or activity and quality targets, take a lot of time away from the few managers that undertake these tasks. Developing tender specifications and undertaking the tendering process takes time. The financial position of the NHS and local authorities will become increasingly stressed over the next two or three years. The NHS funding regime is tight historically and by recent standards, and it is likely this will lead to tough priority setting decisions with services curtailed that many have come to rely on.

As the Bible suggests, prosperity is often followed by austerity: the period to 2008, the seven 'fat' years, may be followed by seven lean years,[1] and suggests a difficult financial period to 2015 at least, and possibly longer! Local authorities have seen a cut in real terms of around 28% over the next four years, much of it frontloaded into 2011–12 and 2012–13. The effects have been dramatic and far-reaching. Many charities and voluntary bodies have or will close, with impacts on children and young people, people with disabilities and older people.

One newspaper report in early August 2011 suggested that the closure of youth centres may have serious repercussions during the summer. A week later, the police station in Tottenham was stormed (London riots: Met Police launch Operation Withern 7 August 2011; http://www.bbc.co.uk/news/uk-england-london-14438109). As an expression of attitudes (not values; i.e. what matters to the local authority), it was a very powerful reminder of the importance of values. What we have is the antithesis of rational planning and financing. Knowing that withdrawal of funds from youth work was likely to exacerbate existing trends,

---

[1] 'And the seven thin and ill favoured kine that came up after them [are] seven years; and the seven empty ears blasted with the east wind shall be seven years of famine' (Genesis 41 : 27).

for whatever reason the local authority reduced dramatically the resources available. Of course, that local authority was not alone. Whether it was inevitable given central government cuts, or an attempt by the local authority to demonstrate the impact, is immaterial. As an expression of values (i.e. what matters to the local authority) it was a very powerful reminder of the importance of values.

The Wanless Reports

The implications of the funding regime were spelt out in 2002 and 2004 by Brian Wanless in his reports to the Chancellor of the Exchequer, in particular the final report on 'Securing good health for the whole population' (Wanless, 2004). Wanless considered the future of the NHS carefully and developed three scenarios that might reflect what could happen over 20 years to 2022. They were:

- Scenario 1: solid progress;
- Scenario 2: slow uptake; and
- Scenario 3: fully engaged.

The report suggests that future health needs and demands will be dependent on the age structure of the population, changes in health status, particularly 'the extent to which improvements in life expectancy are accompanied by improvements in healthy life expectancy'; and the likelihood of health care seeking behaviour. In addition, two further factors were considered: advances in technology and medical advance, and changes to pay and productivity in the health service. These three scenarios were used later (Appleby et al., 2009) to identify the likely funding position for the NHS over the period 2011 to 2016.

Scenario 1: solid progress

In Scenario 1, life expectancy increases with perhaps 5% fewer acute health problems for the elderly, while younger people are more health-aware and seek help for problems that they might not bother with in 2000. Public health targets are met. There is a 3% reduction in smoking for both adults generally and particularly for pregnant women. Teenage birth rates drop and increasing trends in obesity are reversed.[2] The life expectancy gap falls by at least 10%. In other words, 'the solid progress scenario is one of steady improvement with current public health targets met' (Wanless, 2004, p. 38).

Scenario 2: slow uptake

Scenario 2 is essentially the baseline and the most pessimistic of the three. People live longer, but not in good health. Older people particularly will experience long-term illness; and there will be a 10% increase in acute illness. The uptake of new technologies is slow and the benefits of improved IT working are only partially realised.[3] Improvement targets for smoking and diabetes remain the same with no rise in public engagement (Wanless, 2004, pp. 38–39).

---

[2] That is the assumption behind this scenario, but it does not look as good now as it did 10 years ago in relation to improvements in poverty and employment opportunities.

[3] In practice this occurred, as the NPfIT programme was terminated and renegotiated in the summer of 2011.

Scenario 3: fully engaged

In this scenario, people live longer with a smaller proportion of their lives with illness – by 2022 there will have been a 5-year improvement in healthy life. However, the main difference between solid progress and the fully engaged scenarios is a 'dramatic improvement' in public engagement (suggesting, although not spelled out, a greater engagement with public values). Public health improves with a significant reduction in risk factors, such as smoking and obesity. People demand more health (and social care) interventions, so that as health improves, perhaps dramatically, and so does the use by older people of hospital facilities, based on clinical need not age (Wanless, 2004, p. 39).

These scenarios were written roughly 10 years ago, and we are now halfway through the 20-year period that Wanless addressed. We can see that these scenarios contain powerful reflections of values. Life expectancy is given a high profile; confronting health inequalities is critical to a successful health service; tackling smoking and obesity are deemed central; older people are treated for their clinical need, not their age. In particular, a fully engaged public is critical to success. Full engagement means achieving targets through personal actions and accountability; taking responsibility for one's own conduct and that of others; reflecting on prevention and health promotion rather than treatment or care; and achieving productivity by using services sparingly but appropriately. Wanless suggests in Scenario 3 that many younger people will visit GPs more rather than less frequently, often for reassurance. Quality will be the driver; outcomes the measure.

Kings Fund (KF) and Institute for Fiscal Studies (IFS)

The Kings Fund used this agenda as the basis for an important and influential report written jointly with the IFS on the likely funding problems following the crash of 2008 and subsequent events. It is probably true that the next seven years will be very different to the seven years to 2010. Up to 2016–17 we are likely to witness greater financial restraint despite government promises of growth in real terms every year. The National Institute of Economic and Social research (NIESR) predicted in July 2011 that the economy would grow by 1.3% in 2011, and 2% in 2012. This was before the stock market crash in the first week of August 2011. Their prediction for consumer price inflation was that it would fall back from 4.2% in 2011 to 1.9% in 2012; and that the unemployment rate would rise from 7.9% in 2011 to 8.3% in 2012. Productivity performance was considered likely to be disappointing, rising by 1%, on average, over the next few years.

Given this, it is likely that health and social care expenditure will not grow significantly, or at all. Since the inception of the NHS, spending on the NHS has risen around 10-fold in real terms to more than £127 billion. It has also grown as a share of national income, from around 3% to nearly 9% (Appleby et al., 2009). In their report, the Kings Fund and the IFS set out three funding scenarios:

- 'arctic': real funding cuts (–2% for the first three years, –1% for the second three years);
- 'cold': zero real growth for six years; and
- 'tepid': real increase (+2% for the first three years, rising to +3%).

As they point out, 'to put these prospective funding changes in a historical context, there has never been a six-year period of zero real growth in the history of the NHS, and certainly no continuous six-year period of real reductions'. This equates to the most significant cutback to hit the NHS. The most optimistic view of the future, and the one requiring least growth in NHS funding – the 'fully engaged' scenario – assumed, among other things, significant improvements in the population's health as a result mostly of changed behaviours among patients, with a focus on prevention and early intervention, and a productivity improvement of between 2.5 and 3%. The most gloomy scenario –the 'slow uptake' scenario – assumed lower productivity and the continuation of historic trends in population health behaviours. The third scenario – 'solid progress' – differed from the pessimistic view largely on the basis of a steady improvement, with current public health targets met.

All in all, the potential gap in NHS funding, in comparison to Wanless' calculations, is dependent on the position we take on these scenarios. They range from a shortfall of around £4 billion (fully engaged) to a shortfall of nearly £40 billion (slow uptake/arctic) by 2016/17. 'These are equivalent to around 4 per cent and 38 per cent, respectively, of the planned NHS spend in 2010/11' (Appleby et al., 2009). If we consider the graphs reproduced in the report, it is clear where the suggested shortfall of £15 billion to £20 billion came from: an amalgam of the 2013–14 figures for the 'steady progress' scenario and the 'cold' funding stream. 'Gains needed over the next spending review period of around £20 billion under our cold scenario (no real growth in funding) echo indications from NHS Chief Executive David Nicholson of improvements in productivity of around £15–20 billion over this period' (Appleby et al., 2009). Without additional resources, the NHS must find that level of savings for re-investment in new technology, increasing problems of old age and for prevention.

For commissioners this is a momentous challenge. The NHS has not shown itself capable of taking out more than 1%, perhaps at most 2%, in any one year. To be asked to take out 5% year after year is a major assignment. Thresholds for elective care have risen, some treatments are now described as optional, and waiting times have increased, as PCTs (and increasingly CCGs and their allies) seek to restrain spending. Social care is not immune to these savings. Where the NHS may have hoped to off-load care onto community facilities, this is not now possible. While commissioners may want to develop community-oriented facilities and ask social care to meet the cost, the 20%+ reduction in gross local authority spend will now make that impossible. Turning to individual budgets will assist, although they are likely to be severely curtailed; and Health and Well-being Boards will have to work hard to achieve the profiles and savings on an integrative basis.

Health and well-being

Since the advent of the White Paper 'Equity and Excellence: Liberating the NHS' (Department of Health, 2010), there has been a good deal of uncertainty about the future of the NHS (which continues at the time of writing). One possibility is that the NHS and other agencies will be remodelled into a number of care streams based on the care pathway approach. While we do not know what will happen, the change to a pathways model may not provide the robustness that values-based commissioning requires, but at the same time offers opportunities for values to be brought centre stage. The diagram here (Figure 4.1) is overly simple, but suggests the concentration or specialisation that may occur.

The strategic approach adopted here suggests that acute hospitals, for example, will be expected to concentrate on treating acute illness and leave everything else to other agencies. On the other hand, the move towards integration may mean that acute hospitals become 'providers of everything'. Feedback loops need to be included in the diagram, but the general tenor is clear. Many PCTs have placed an emphasis on tackling health inequalities through

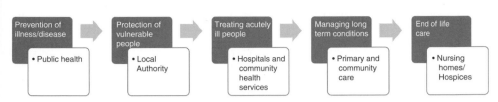

Figure 4.1 Existing specialisation that may develop further.

working with local authorities in their area that are part of the Spearhead group. Although targets were generally no longer the government's favourite approach (until November 2011, when the Secretary of State re-introduced them), many will stay in one form or another, often as desired outcomes, or as modified Public Service Agreement (PSA) targets. It is likely that the new public health service will have similar population outcome targets. A national health inequalities PSA target was set in 2001 with the aim of reducing inequalities in infant mortality and life expectancy by 2010. Updated in 2004, it was supported by two more detailed objectives around infant mortality and life expectancy (see Chapter 6).

A recent NAO Report (2010) highlighted progress made on the relevant PSA targets. One of the NAO recommendations was that greater investment (not less) is necessary, if the NHS is to help tackle health inequalities now in the future, a recommendation that was also echoed by the Marmot Review (2010). The important point to consider is what, from a values-based commissioning perspective, would be the right direction to take in developing Wanless' 'fully engaged' scenario.

A group of values that has gained in operative momentum over the previous 10 years concerns prevention and health promotion. Although health promotion has been funded by the NHS for the previous 30 years or so, it is only in the last 10 years that it has had wider support. There are a number of reasons for the delay in achieving some traction. First, many senior managers have been, and frankly remain, sceptical of the cost–benefit of health promotion. This is despite good evidence of success in limited areas. Second, there has never been enough money to justify spending large sums on prevention or health promotion when there are other priorities on which the money could be spent; and third, until recently, the priorities of the NHS have been about targets in acute care, not targets for well-being and prevention of illness.

As it happens, the last five years or so have seen a resurgence of interest in health promotion and mental well-being. This is less concerned about preventing mental illness, although that is one important part of it. Mental well-being is for everyone. So the new paradigm suggests a 'three-cornered hat': promoting mental well-being for all; preventing mental health problems for those at risk; and assisting those with living in recovery to the best well-being possible. Another reason is the realisation that this is a shared endeavour between health and social care, and that this might act as a catalyst for integrative commissioning, or an amalgamation of functions through the role of Health and Well-being Boards. Well-being becomes the glue that holds health and social care together.

By placing a premium on health and well-being we are demonstrating the espoused values of the NHS and social care (Argyris and Schon, 1978). Refracting evidence through a wide-angle values lens offers the opportunity to coalesce population perspectives, community views, group concerns with individual values in order to tackle the Wanless agenda. We need to bring together economics, ethics, equalities and evidence under the rubric of values. There are two main economic reasons for investing in health promotion and prevention: improved mental and physical health (i.e. reduced illness) leads to NHS and social care savings; and improved mental well-being leads to savings in other areas of health and social care. As the Royal College of Psychiatrists has noted:

- People with mental disorder smoke almost half of all tobacco consumed and account for almost half of all smoking-related deaths.
- Depression doubles the risk of developing coronary heart disease.
- People with two or more long-term physical illnesses have a sevenfold greater risk of depression.
- Children from the poorest households have a threefold greater risk of mental illness than children from the richest household (Royal College of Psychiastrists, 2010).

Wanless again: exploring the link with full engagement

The 'fully engaged' scenario requires a 'dramatic improvement' in public engagement. Public health improves with a significant reduction in risk factors such as smoking and obesity. People will, Wanless argued, demand more health (and social care) interventions so that as health improves, perhaps dramatically, so does the use of hospital facilities by older people, based on clinical need not age, and so does the use of GP services by younger people as much for reassurance as anything else.

Physical health and mental health are much more entangled than is generally realised. For example, the costs to the NHS per person between the ages of 10 and 28 are nearly nine times higher among those who had conduct disorders than among those with no conduct problems at this age. Effective evidence-based interventions can reduce illness and NHS costs in the short term and over the life course. Between 25% and 50% of adult mental disorders are potentially preventable with treatment during childhood and adolescence (Kim-Cohen *et al.*, 2003). Good evidence-based interventions can result in improved educational and psycho-social outcomes; and improved mental well-being leads to savings in a number of areas, such as reduced drinking or lowered rates of coronary heart disease (CHD).

Ethical and values-based arguments for these interventions are compelling. There is a need for commissioning that understands the value of relationships, and builds interpersonal awareness and interdependence within connected communities. Emphasising rights and responsibilities with individual and community capacities provides the context for a social commissioning. A growing body of evidence on the social determinants of health, such as the Marmot Review, demonstrates that preventive and health promoting strategies will achieve a greater social cohesion while encouraging individual responsibility for personal health and community well-being (Marmot, 2010; Wilkinson and Pickett, 2009). Poor mental well-being is both a cause and a consequence of health and social inequalities (Friedli, 2009).

There is now strong evidence that mental health and physical health are intimately inter-related (see for example Royal College of Psychiatrists, 2010; Foresight Report, 2009). Good mental well-being can: increase life expectancy, provide protection from coronary heart disease and improve health outcomes more generally; reduce risks to health by influencing positive behaviours; and influence the social determinants of health. These improvements lead on to improved educational attainment, safer communities with less crime, improved productivity and employment retention, and reduced sickness absence from work (Newbigging and Heginbotham, 2010).

Commissioning for well-being requires an understanding of individual and community reliance and the factors that enable individuals and communities to remain healthy, independent and interdependent. In turn this means understanding diversity and difference, local health and social care inequalities, and insists that individual and groups with special needs and aspirations have a voice. To achieve the best from such a programme demands opportunities in all public services (and publicly *funded* services) to promote physical and mental well-being, including creating supportive environments in homes, schools, workplaces, shopping areas, and neighbourhood centres.

There is some evidence that by implementing those interventions that we know will work, there will be a cumulative effect of improved well-being and reduced costs. One project may have an impact, but 2 or 3 or 5 or 10 will make a much bigger cumulative difference. Many present commissioners are not grasping this opportunity, either because they do not believe the savings that might accrue, or because they have little time to investigate the benefits, or because they simply have a prejudice against health and well-being interventions. Health and Well-being Boards will have the chance to address these attitudes (and values) assertively and increasingly over the next three years or so. The evidence for what works is persuasive.

Evidence and outcomes

One of the most important factors in using evidence robustly and assertively is in relation to outcomes. Outcomes-led commissioning draws heavily on values-based practice. The outcomes of an intervention are of two sorts: the outcome of the treatment or other action taken, which we assume uses evidence-based medicine and social care; and the expectations of the patient or service user. Thus the outcome is a compound of what we know, or think we know, about the treatment itself, its risks and benefits (and which we assume has been discussed with the patient by the treating clinicians), and the patient's acceptance of those risks; and the prospective or anticipated results that the patient desires from the treatment (Figure 4.2).

Both sets of information have individual and collective components. There is an individual aspect (the patient in discussion with the clinicians about what works, the risks, individual values and expectations, and so on) and there is a collective voice (the group, or community) concerning evidence and values.

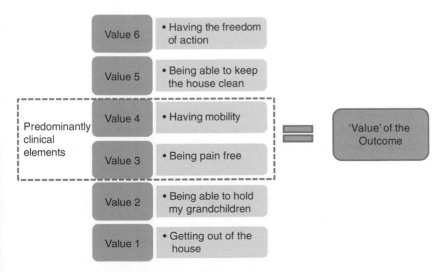

Figure 4.2 Creating an outcome from the values of the patient or service user.

The value of the agreed and adopted approach is the value, expressed as an outcome, of recognising and acting upon the set of values that the patient or service user considers important. While that is what matters to health and social care in the UK, it is far from universal. In some jurisdictions the value of the outcome is that which is determined by the treatment evidence alone. In the UK the 'value' of the outcome draws on the expected utility – on the expected values – of the patient. In Figure 4.2, the 'value' of the outcome of a hip replacement operation is predicated on achieving the 'values' on the left-hand side.

Being able to live pain-free, or being able to hold her grandchildren, are the values that made the patient agree to the hip replacement in the first place. While the technical and clinical features of the operation were important (she wanted it to be successful), many (if not most) of them were too technical and possibly beyond her understanding. She placed her confidence in the surgeon, anaesthetist, junior doctors, theatre nurses and theatre manager to know what they were doing! However, what mattered to her very much were the values described. Values-based practice accords these values as great an importance as the evidence.

Evidence-based medicine; values-based practice

The key point about V-BP is that it is the corollary not the antithesis of E-BM. Good practice ensures that evidence is refracted through the lens of values. We need to know values, not because it changes the evidence, but because it changes the way we read or interpret the evidence.

Case example: Rheumatoid Arthritis

An example of the importance of values in medicine is provided by the differences in approach of clinicians and patients with rheumatoid arthritis. Clinicians tend to be concerned with a description of the way a loss or change of function occurs and with its clinical amelioration (a medical model focusing on disease processes); patients tend to be concerned with the implications and consequences of drug toxicity (Fraenkel et al., 2004; Goodacre and Goodacre, 2004) or loss of function for activities of daily living; in other words, with the 'illness' effects. As personalisation develops in medicine and in social care the attitudes of both patients and service users, and of clinicians, will necessarily change, with much greater involvement of patients in determining the outcomes appropriate for them as well as in the objectives of clinical research (see also Chapter 5 on patient and service user engagement; Birrell et al., 2011).

One reason for this is the development of personalised biologic therapies for rheumatoid arthritis. As monoclonal antibody therapies proliferate, attention to the way they work with individual patients will be indispensable. Individual values, for example on tolerance of pain, which will vary noticeably from one patient to another, will affect the type and dose of treatment given. 'In order to maximise their benefit : risk ratios and to minimise later joint damage . . .', it will be necessary to have predictors of the efficacy of the drugs used and the patients' attitude to their consequences (Isaacs and Ferraccioli, 2010).

As important is the way that clinicians and patients recognise the outcomes of care. Many physicians suggest that the aetiology of functional disorder is paramount and work hard to recognise and describe symptoms and complications, and to seek treatments that minimise progressive harms. Conversely, patients are concerned less with describing the impact on their joints than in the implications for their activities of daily life, such as cooking, cleanliness, or personal hygiene. For instance, in reviewing the Health Assessment Questionnaire Disability Index (HAQ-DI; the most widely used measure of function in rheumatoid arthritis) in order to enhance the incorporation of patients' views in outcome assessment, individualised questionnaires measuring importance gave complementary importance to measures of disability (Seror et al., 2010). Although the HAQ contained approximately 70% of the items patients suggested proactively should be included, *there was relatively little correlation with individual anxieties* (Hewlett et al., 2001) (my emphasis).

Equal partnerships between clinicians and patients can cover the whole clinical programme or pathway, not just parts of it, and involve experiential and mutual learning, openness, and respect, which assist in overcoming stereotypes and tensions. These differences may be ameliorated by clinician–patient interactions that recognise competing values at play and give greater weight to patient preferences or to those aspects of treatment outcomes that truly reflect the obstacles patients surmount in day-to-day activity. Despite fears that clinicians 'misinterpret the relevance of disability for the patient' (Hewlett et al., 2001), engaging patient values gives patients greater say and improves research programme objectives. Patients are increasingly involved actively in responsive research and progressively more as research partners (Abma et al., 2009; de Wit et al., 2011). As this occurs, more and more patient values become built into the evidence; and progressively the evidence reflects those values.

Evidence-based practice

'Evidence-based medicine ... is the conscientious, explicit and judicious use of current best evidence in making decisions about the care of individual patients. The practice of evidence-based medicine means integrating individual clinical expertise with the best available external clinical evidence from systematic research' (Sackett, 1997). Evidence-based practices are interventions for which there is scientific evidence showing consistent improvement in client outcomes. However, there have been many examples where evidence is not used routinely, especially in psychiatry and other disciplines that, paradoxically, rely heavily on values.

Despite extensive evidence and agreement on what constitutes effective mental health practice for persons with severe mental illness, clinicians do not 'provide evidence-based practices to the great majority of their clients with these illnesses' (Drake *et al.*, 2001). Psychiatry in particular demands a wider relationship with a range of stakeholders and positions, given the contentious nature of much treatment. For example (see Chapter 7), many patients want to 'de-medicalise' mental health treatment by replacing current packages of care with alternative complementary treatments (NHS Confederation, 2011).

Values that may inform evidence must be treated carefully but openly (Sackett *et al.*, 2000). Patient values are shaped by many factors, not least family narratives and discussions over many years, providing a complex yet balanced understanding of family medical histories (Lindenmeyer *et al.*, 2011). The last 10 years, however, have seen much greater emphasis on evidence and latterly on values. A tension exists between 'the "scientific" practice of medicine that is epistemically and ethically incompatible with medical decision making based on human experiences, preferences and values' (Cronje and Fullan, 2003) which has been described as a 'dissonance' between 'objective measurement ... and ... clinical judgment' (Greenhalgh, 1999, p. 323 quoted in Cronje and Fullan, 2003). More importantly, EBM offers the promise of a more 'rational' discourse and places an emphasis on truth, validity and rationality.

An example of this is shown in variations of 'vertical equity', where no one treatment for similar conditions stands out as preferable (Heginbotham *et al.*, 1992). Coronary Artery Bypass Graft (CABG) and Percutaneous Coronary Intervention (CPI) (usually referred to as coronary angioplasty) are typical examples, especially where non-surgical options are also available (Wennberg *et al.*, 2008), and substantial differences in rates of as much as 10-fold for CABG and PCI have been reported (Centre for the Evaluative Clinical Sciences, 2005). As Appleby and colleagues report (Appleby *et al.*, 2011, pp. 22–24), although case-mix differences may contribute to the variations described, and patient preferences might have a role to play, it is 'unlikely that such choices vary as sharply at the level of PCTs as do the surgical ratios'. More importantly, they suggest that there are two main reasons in the literature. The first is the uncertainty about who will benefit from treatments; but more importantly it is because clinicians fail accurately to 'understand patients' values and preferences' (Bursztajn *et al.*, 1990). In fact, patients will often opt to wait or take the least-invasive route rather than undertake potentially dangerous surgery.

Public health, for example, has sought to improve the scientific standards for evidence underlying interventions and has begun to question common assumptions about the types of evidence required to demonstrate the efficacy and effectiveness of public health interventions. Over time, this led to an increase in the use of RCTs in order to improve the evidence available, and in turn this fuelled the quality standards of clinical research. Subsequently, there has been a realisation that the RCT is not the only way in which evidence can be gathered, and that patient preferences and demands have validity as long as they are captured in a rigorous way.

Values-based practice potentially undermines this promise by interposing patient and service user experiences, values and preferences. In practice this is much less of a problem than it might seem at first, but only if we (and clinicians especially) allow a broader conception of 'rational' than is usually used in medicine. The medical literature demonstrates an equivocal attitude which suggests a 'collective need to better integrate scientific quantitative data ... and the art of human judgment ... into a common definition of "rational" medical practice' (Cronje and Fullan, 2003). In other words, to be 'rational' we must have both the biological or medical facts as best as we can get them and the values of those to whom the facts will be applied.

Many advocates of E-BP are aware of the need to integrate patients into the clinical decision-making process (see for example Coulter and Collins, 2011). Patients' preferences are critical to research and were included when E-BM was first developed (Haynes *et al.*, 2002) and others have suggested that patients' and service users' values can 'affect the balance' between the likely treatment options and the involvement of the patient. However, this does not engage patients honestly and openly in a meaningful debate, or as full and autonomous citizens (Sackett *et al.*, 2000); nor does it ensure their values are taken into account other than in the marginal space of uncertainty left over once the majority of the clinical space has been colonised by medical options over which there is no discussion. Haynes argues that the scope of clinical expertise is limited, as shown in Figure 4.3.

If the rationality model is valuable it must be a model of rationality that by definition includes patient and service user values alongside a careful assessment of the evidence of effectiveness and outcomes of the treatment options. Only by properly bringing the E-BP and V-BP together can the full benefits be realised for the clinician as much as the patient. There is no condition–treatment pair that does not demand a proper balance of patients' values and preferences and clinical evidence and judgement. Some situations are more biological than others – in certain sorts of surgery, for example – and some have a much larger values base – such as in psychiatry. However, all have the two components which require a form of rationality that enables them to be both extant and engaged.

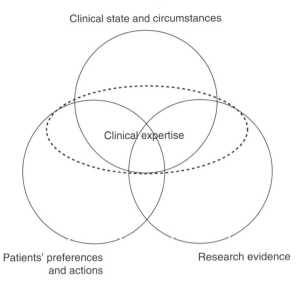

Clinical state and circumstances

Clinical expertise

Patients' preferences
and actions

Research evidence

Figure 4.3 From Haynes *et al.*, (2002, *British Medical Journal*), with permission from the author.

To meet this requirement, Cronje and Fullan suggest a rationality structure based on work by Brown (1990) and Habermas (1984). In this they posit an integrated process of human judgement that relies on 'social validation, dynamic processes, freedom from coercion and inclusivity of all stakeholders'. In achieving the necessary balance they accept that it is impossible for an individual patient, 'trapped within her own subjectivity, to know for certain that her judgments are sound or defensible' (Cronje and Fullan, 2003). Any judgement must convince others, even one that proposes treatment options for which there may be little or no evidence, or where narratives need to be heard (Little *et al.*, 1999). Therefore, this is a *social* rationality rather than a medical or rule driven rationality, which relies on narrative to understand the options available.

An alternative to this is that proposed by Seedhouse (2005). 'Values-based decision-making' proposes and describes a standard computerised model with elements that can be amended or weighted depending on the matter at hand. While this has advantages once the model has been revised for a particular purpose, a full discussion is beyond the scope of this book. However, there are clear similarities between values-based decision-making and values-based commissioning, notably but not exclusively that values *become* evidence, or at any rate affect the evidence, if handled correctly. There may be more appropriate ways of capturing all that is needed for values-based practice, but it is important that values are engaged.

Conclusion

Evidence-based practice is the other half-field that complements values-based practice. By bringing evidence and values into contention we can ensure both aspects are fully engaged and contribute to making decisions about priorities and resource allocation. By bringing evidence and values together, we develop a form of narrative rationality that recognises both the importance of good evidence, and the need for human judgement.

Chapter 5

Patient and public involvement

Background remarks

Community engagement is as important for values-based practice as the process of agreeing or dissenting about the values themselves. Only by understanding values will it be possible to engage in a proper discussion about values and get to a point of dissensus. Knowing the values and aspirations of patients and service users is a critical feature of the process. Unfortunately, in the past, commissioners have not often acted responsibly to truly understand values in a way that enables a genuine debate. This is made more difficult by the requirements of the 'strong' or 'thick' system of values-based understanding.

Learning the values of one individual or a small group of defined service users is relatively easy; obtaining a composite set of values from sets of users across an area, supplemented by the values of groups of professional commissioning staff, Health and Well-being Boards, and the public, will be immensely more difficult. Many GPs involved in commissioning are likely to be impatient to get some results, especially because of the delays in legislation, but also because of the financial situation that requires a 'decent minimum' set of service responses. However, in its way, this offers scope for a wider process that can provide a set of values to ensure all opportunities for values-based commissioning are taken.

If we consider the need for decisions on service pathways and profiles to ensure that we can live within the budgets available, there are four levels of action and understanding, as follows.

- At a population level, there is a need for an outcomes-led approach that builds on values of the population to make large-scale changes that are both cost effective and acceptable to the majority. These may not be acceptable to all, but in the main will ensure that all patients get the right elements of a service.
- At a community level, there may be specific concerns that affect that community (or local authority, or PCT cluster area). Most of these concerns will be centred on more specific circumstances locally – a proposed new hospital, for example, or the cessation of a well-known service. These concerns require values-based consideration, but will be more localised, may engage quite diverse sections of the community depending on the issue, and will be more or less contentious.
- At a group level, there will be more immediate and localised matters. A group of people with Type II diabetes, for example, will have a number of critical but similar issues to debate, even though their values and those of the commissioners may diverge considerably.
- Finally, at the individual level, the use of values-based commissioning, especially for 'hard cases', will be of real importance to the individual. In such cases it may be necessary to

ensure that the values of the individual are considered in the light of discussions with the community and/or the group. For example, a person with diabetes may want a hospital service to be available, when the commissioners are trying hard to develop community services with very little hospital care. The community group may have agreed in general with this direction of travel, and the patient group will have suggested that this is the most reasonable approach, but even so, the individual, perhaps for good reasons, wants to have access to a hospital service.

Each level demands a different process based on:

- the outcomes that the level can deal with adequately; and
- the way in which the engagement process can be run.

Localism

To add to the complexity, the Localism Act 2011 allows a number of changes to the consultation process on local authority services (Localism goes to the Lords, 2011); the Spearhead Group of local authorities, supported by the Association of Public Health Observatories (APHO) and Department of Health (DH) websites, offers a number of local authority-assisted interventions aimed at improving overall life expectancy; and the raft of White Papers on health suggest the need for effective consultation. A recent consultation exercise by Department of Communities and Local Government (DCLG) on the 'Community Right to Challenge' was about the opportunity for community and voluntary bodies, parish councils and authority employees to bid to take over the running of local authority services (DCLG, 2011).

Many local authorities recognise the role that some groups can play in designing and delivering local services, providing new ideas, a deeper and often better understanding of service users' needs, and offering good value for taxpayers' money. The Localism Act 2011 will give these groups the chance to bring proposals about running a service to the local council and require it to give them proper consideration. How this will impact on health and well-being is unclear, although it is fascinating that it will become law more or less at the same time that CCGs take on health service commissioning. Undoubtedly it will strengthen values-based commissioning, and the values of communities and local groups will take on a new importance.

The 'Community Right to Challenge' includes opportunities for voluntary groups to express an interest in running council services, even if these services presently generate a surplus. Although there has been a strongly statist approach to local government services in the recent past, the Labour Party approach to the Localism Act will undoubtedly change, as will the Coalition government's approach to the 'Big Society'. That the Labour Party will become more accommodating and attenuate their attack that the rhetoric of 'localism' is at odds with the front-loaded cuts that face many local authorities. On the other hand, the Coalition may temper its attitude towards localism; localism must mean more than dismantling local services and putting faith in volunteers to pick up the pieces.

Localism must serve more than those with the loudest voices, the most strident views, and the deepest pockets. Overall, a balance will need to be struck between driving power down to communities, and retaining the facility to deliver strategic national infrastructure such as new nuclear power stations. By and large, local government staff and others of a statist mindset need to move beyond the 'state' and find ways to engage broader sections of society in shaping their neighbourhoods and empowering people.

What is unclear is the extent to which this Act will be used to develop genuinely robust consultation and alternative service elements for Health and Well-being Boards, and for public health, especially as one of the critical aspects of the Localism Act is housing. Those component parts of local government may not be immune to the implications of the Act. Local Councils may run with new and quite different interpretations of what consultation means, and assume that the purpose of localism is to create a multi-layered interpretation. A Cooperative Councils Network (launched in Rochdale on 15 July 2011), set up to tap into the mutualism and cooperative systems that run deep in the history of the left in the UK (Reed, 2011) draws inspiration from the values of fairness, accountability and responsibility. It offers a communities approach to values, and to understanding the way that broad values shape services, and within which individual and group values can operate.

Such a development of mutualism and cooperativeness also provides scope for community-led commissioning, by using community engagement techniques and a programme of change management. This will encourage a joined up, user-led approach to health, housing and social care services and thus to integration of health, housing, education and social service delivery (Turning Point, 2011). It provides a form of values-based process, rooted in engaging sections of the community to develop 'connected care', essentially a way in which health, social care, education, housing and other key elements of local services can be constructed differently in an overlapping, intersecting, efficient and economical way.

Community engagement

Engaging communities and groups of users is a fraught process that has been done tolerably well in some places and very badly in others. The basic problem is twofold: many PCTs have not held strong views about the importance of values and therefore have not seen deep engagement processes as necessary; and paradoxically, the decisions about care have often been seen as urgent, or at least as urgent enough that there is too little time to engage a community meaningfully. The implication is that many PCTs have paid lip service to genuine community engagement and, where possible, have used short cuts and overly simple processes that will not get to the heart of the problem.

Community engagement should be a genuine, real attempt to understand the needs of the community in a way that engages the core of the community (see Figure 5.1). This does not mean the 'leaders' whoever they are, but the 'real' people, those who often do not have a voice that is heard, but who form the basis of community views. However, the approach will vary depending on a number of factors:

- Which level are we concerned to tackle?
- Which issue do we want to understand?
- How much money or other resources do we have at our disposal?
- When do we have to make a decision on the resource allocation question?

As we tease out the answer to these questions, we begin to see the need for a composite and comprehensive policy that achieves the objective of our quest: to understand the values and the interplay of values of the group, or community or population that we have targeted.

The critical point is that we are concerned with values, not with the decisions on resources or organisation, important as those are. The aim of values-based commissioning is to establish a community engagement programme that learns from the service users either

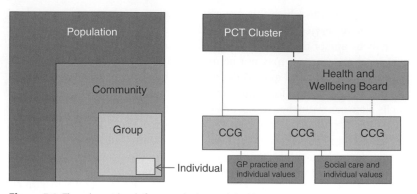

Figure 5.1 The relevant levels for consultation and decision.

from them alone or in dialogue with professional staff and others. As we saw in Chapter 1, there is a need to consider whether to develop a weak system that goes only so far in detailing the values of the group, community or population, or whether to develop a strong process that recognises the importance of a wider and deeper understanding of values that will stand the process in good stead.

The process can be either at each level separately or in a combination. CCGs (as described at summer 2011) will have the main responsibility to develop group values that can be used to examine the priorities for individual services, and we can assume that PCT clusters will have the main responsibility for the population level. Even though PCT clusters are relatively small, in some cases they have a substantial population and spend: Greater Manchester has a population of 2,646,500 and a spend of £4657 million (at one end of the spectrum) to Cumbria with a population of 509,000 and a spend of £811 million (at the other) (all figures at 2011–2012). With four super-regions it is likely that PCT clusters will act to ensure that population perspectives are derived at that level, although it is doubtful if they will do anything such as community engagement. That is likely to be left to local government and the CCGs.

As we have seen, understanding values is not a process that has been attempted frequently. The 'standard' community engagement processes have been used to understand the attitude of Black and minority ethnic communities in relation to drugs, or the approach that a group of people in a community might have towards a limited list marginal priorities list, or perhaps as a research tool for a citizens' jury. None of these have attempted to extract the fundamental values that apply to the decisions that are taken. Of course, there is some overlap between the levels, but this will at times be confusing.

Values can be ascertained using all the standard mechanisms amended or adjusted to elicit values rather than other objectives. For example, the citizens' jury (see Chapter 8 for a list of references to Citizens Juries and other mechanisms of engagement) can be used to decide on the balance between competing priorities, but may also be used explicitly to identify the values that the members of the jury bring to the decisions. Similarly, focus groups may be used to obtain views about the status of different health or social care initiatives, but may also be used carefully to understand the values that the members bring.

Community engagement is used extensively in relation to public health need and practice with a specific focus on reducing health inequalities and improving well-being. This has used a variety of approaches including neighbourhood forums, citizen juries, collaborative methodologies and health or social care champions. All of these can be used to generate values, but were not set up with that in mind. Although many approaches have been used, a number of factors prevent them being effective. These include:

- the culture and attitude of statutory agencies;
- the dominance of professional elites and their cultures;
- competing priorities within the statutory agencies;
- the skills and abilities of staff; and
- the capacity and willingness of service users and the public. (Pickin *et al.*, 2002, quoted in NICE, 2008)

In practice, the involvement of patients, service users and carers in determining values is difficult, but it is rewarding as it carries the opportunity to have a meaningful and much deeper conversation between service users and professional commissioners (GPs, nurses, managers, etc.). As Popay (2006) has shown, there is a welcome improvement in service, social capital and empowerment, and health outcomes in moving from informing, through consultation and co-production, towards delegated power and community control. The latter two may not be possible or desirable in all cases, but in some services where personal budgets (in health or social care) are available, such outcomes may be achievable. From a V-BC perspective, we are interested in achieving the best care and support from health and social care with the resources available to meet the needs, wishes, aspirations and (especially) the values of service users, and which will be used as effectively as possible. This can be achieved by improving the understanding of values and their use through a process of greater community control (as noted in Figure 5.2). Not only do health outcomes improve, but a range of service and intermediate social outcomes do too.

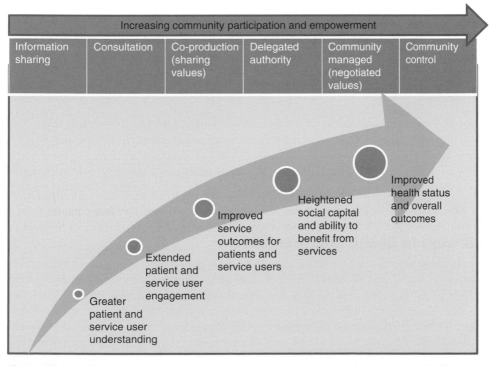

Figure 5.2 Increasing community participation leads to improved outcomes and ever-increasing health status.

Values-based community engagement demands different processes to those attempts to define the objectives of service development or health improvement. While joint strategic needs assessment (JSNA) is a critical (and values-based) programme, it does not directly assist in determining the values that need to be considered for commissioning. JSNA depends on but does not elucidate values. Differing levels of and approaches to community engagement are underpinned by differing value systems and it is thus necessary to clarify what we want to know.

Community engagement has a number of methodological problems (NICE, 2008). There is no single definition of either 'community' or 'engagement'; no two definitions are the same. More importantly, the approach to community engagement has rarely been the subject of research which has concentrated on the outcomes of the process rather than the process itself. Much of the community engagement that has been evaluated is understandably not cost-effective, or the cost-effectiveness calculations can be overturned by minor changes to certain assumptions (Knapp *et al.*, 2010). This is true of collaborative methodology, health trainers and citizens' juries (NICE, 2008, p. 16). In practice, there are four important interlocking themes: setting up the projects correctly; establishing an infrastructure; approaches to encourage and support community engagement; and evaluation of the project.

In reviewing the NICE Guidelines it is worth noting certain key elements of the recommendations. For instance, action in relation to Recommendation 3 suggests that those running a project should:

- encourage local people to help identify priorities;
- consider diversity training and raise cultural awareness;
- encourage all communities to express their opinions (regardless about whether they disagree with national, regional or local policy);
- give weight to the views of local people when decisions affecting them are taken; and
- manage conflict between and within communities, and the agencies that serve them.

Although these suggestions do not directly address values-based commissioning, they do act as warnings about significant aspects of community engagement. In Recommendation 4 there is a call to identify how power is distributed and to 'negotiate and agree . . . how power should be shared and distributed'. Making all parties aware of the importance of community involvement and in particular the importance of diversity and difference is another important step (NICE, 2008).

Pathways to health improvement

What matters, however, is how we build on this advice to develop a values-based system. The evidence is sketchy, but suggests that we need to have a composite process that draws from the four levels and examines the way that values are used by different groups. Black and minority ethnic groups will have differing values based on ethnicity, country of origin, culture, faith and religion and their present place of residence. Some of their values will be common to the majority, some will be very different. Similarly, older people, or lesbian and

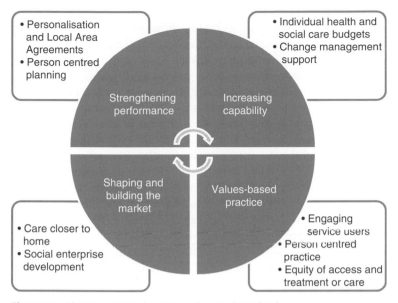

Figure 5.3 Obtaining values depends on the population level.

gay or disabled people, will have some similar and some different values. Some of these values may seem odd to another group, for example the professional staff of services, but careful assessment will demonstrate how they have arisen and why they matter. No individual's values are better than anyone else's. They differ, and that difference must be used to throw light on the way that health and social care is managed (Figure 5.3).

The four levels of values-based practice need to be brought together into an effective programme that builds on the right mix of different components. To be genuinely effective requires that commissioners consider the values that they will need for the decisions that they have to take. If a 'weak' system is used it will be easier initially and much harder later to get patients and service users to engage meaningfully. Conversely, using a 'strong' system will take time at the beginning but save time later.

Engaging with communities: step change and discontinuity

One of the most difficult things to do is relate commissioner perspectives to community situations where there are discontinuities in either the behaviour of the patient or service user, or in the system that is provided. This is especially true of values-based decisions.

Take one example. A woman takes her eight-year-old to school and then goes to work half an hour's travel time from the school. At 11.30 a.m. the school rings her to say that her child has fallen in the playground and is now in the sick bay. He seems to be alright and there is no immediate reason for serious concern, but the school would like the mother, or another person, to call and collect the child and take him to A&E. The mother is worried that leaving work at 11.45 to go to the school will lead to difficulties with her employer. When this happened before she was warned that a repeat might lead to her being sacked, or at least losing a day's pay. She rings the A&E and asks whether it will be possible to bring her son later in the day. The casualty registrar says that A&E is quiet at the moment and that he will be seen straight away if she brings him now, but at 5 p.m. it may be a different story and she may have to wait a long time. What does she do? What whole values come into play?

The mother is the key person in the story given there is no other person able or willing to take her son to hospital. Her values include two possibly contradictory principles: she has a strong work ethic and is mortified that her employer might sack her for taking time to deal with her son; but the employer's approach is worrying and causes her real anxiety. Her son appears alright and while she is a good mother it sounds as though he can wait until 5 p.m. However, at 5 p.m. the A&E may be very busy and it is always possible that a road traffic accident or some other event might make it worse. Guiding the mother to the correct decision is challenging.

On one level this is a values-based conflict. The school would like the mother to collect the son, even though there is probably nothing seriously wrong with him, and take him to A&E where there are staff available. But the mother has her work ethic, her values, and does not perceive that she is needed immediately, especially as she will not be able to tell a convincing story at work as her son is not 'at death's door'. The mother will decide and the school will have to accept that the son will stay in the sick bay until he recovers sufficiently, or will be collected by his mother to take him to A&E at 5 p.m. This will of course depend on whether he deteriorates and his condition becomes urgent. In this case, the school may call an ambulance and take the matter out of the mother's hands.

Negotiating value differences in these circumstances will be difficult. There is not a lot of time; the school teacher, A&E clinician and the mother are in different places physically; and the only means of communication is on the telephone. Under other circumstances when the situation may arise regularly, spending some time to agree to differ or to come to an understanding about when and under what circumstances the mother should go to the school would be beneficial. On another level, this is a classic situation that may be modelled by the use of catastrophe theory. Catastrophe theory is a mathematical theory that explains the observation that small incremental changes in the value of a variable in a natural system can lead to sudden large changes in the state of the system (Last, 2006).[1] The best-known, everyday example is the change in the state of water from solid (ice) to liquid (water) to gas (steam); another example is the unpredictable timing and scale of a landslide. The same processes occur in health systems, including certain stages in the process of carcinogenesis and spread of cancer, in gene frequencies in populations, and in epidemiological science such as the appearance and disappearance of epidemics.

The word 'catastrophe' with its suggestion that the outcome is always undesirable may have been an unhappy choice to describe this process. While this is certainly the case in the rapid onset of many epidemics, the same mathematical process operates in reverse when an epidemic or epidemic disease virtually disappears quite suddenly from a population. This happens when the balance of susceptible and immune individuals shifts from the proportion required to sustain an epidemic to a marginally smaller proportion where the probability of

---

[1] Catastrophe theory began with the work of the French mathematician René Thom in the 1960s, followed by Christopher Zeeman in the 1970s (Zeeman, 1977), and considers the way that small changes in certain parameters of a non-linear system can cause equilibria to appear or disappear, or to change from attracting to repelling and vice versa, leading to large and sudden changes of the behaviour of the system (Wikipedia, accessed 10 August 2011).

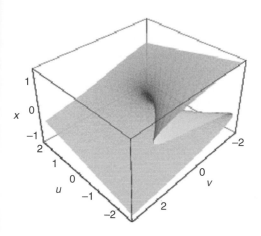

Figure 5.4 The cusp catastrophe.

transmission of an infectious agent to a susceptible host falls below the critical level required to sustain the epidemic (Last, 2006).

The most helpful use of a catastrophe theory is in predicting and managing complex situations. The cusp catastrophe, the most useful for our purposes, is shown in Figure 5.4. This model has a number of uses. Let us consider a political demonstration. During the demonstration the police recognise that if pushed too far, the group may become violent. By forcing them into a smaller and smaller space, there is a point when the group dynamics get to the point of discontinuity and 'drops' to the lower level, exciting a riot. Conversely, if the folk are led around the discontinuity they could be brought to the new state without rioting. Another example might be from the stock exchange. In this case we get more distinct transitions from a normal day to either a 'bear' market with panic selling, or a 'bull' market with sudden buying. Either can be modelled well using the cusp catastrophe.

In our case of the mother called to collect her son, there are three options. The first is to leave the mother, having discussed the position and decided it is not worth pursuing. A second option is to seek to lead her round the discontinuity onto the lower level, which corresponds to a different set of behaviours.

By manipulating the information available (the extent of injury to the son; the mother's values about work) it may be possible to negotiate a compromise for her to collect her son, perhaps in the early afternoon. The third possibility is to force the issue by talking up the injury and making her understand her responsibility to him (and incidentally to the NHS). This drives the trajectory towards the bifurcation and towards a place where the result is unstable, leading her to a sudden behaviour change – a realisation that she must after all attend to her son. This process can be used in other situations of values conflict, such as human resources, mental health treatment (without using powers under the Act), and so on. Using catastrophe theory enables us to see the implications of our values and the way that sudden and apparently unpredictable changes can occur.

Engaging minority groups

Health and social care organisations need to understand the values and culture that under-pins and contextualises minority values, whether those are of Black and minority ethnic communities, disabled people, the values of gay and lesbian groups, and so on. These have and will continue to change so that no previous research or values statement is a reliable guide to how individuals or communities think at present. Many PCTs have a narrow view of minority communities' values. Although Black groups may have many values that are the same or similar to White or other minority ethnic groups, there will be some differences, while significant differences may be apparent in the values or attitudes of a small minority of Black people. Two critical issues need to be recognised. First, the values and approaches of some people, such as those of south Asian heritage, will be shaped largely by differences in faith and religion and their inherent understandings of the way the world works; and second, the issues of race are often overshadowed by income deprivation, educational attainment or lack of work opportunities.

Describing minority communities by focusing on ethnicity misses a powerful point about the range, scope and nature of minorities. The Equalities Act 2010 sets out nine categories, known as 'protected characteristics' on which discrimination is outlawed: age, gender (sex), ethnicity (race), sexual orientation, gender reassignment, faith or religion, disability, marriage and civil partnership, and pregnancy and maternity. Ensuring that the values of all those groups and communities is considered fully is a challenge for CCGs and Health and Well-being Boards. While we can know some of their values some of the time, we cannot, without careful and frequent analysis, understand the implications. For example, the 'Count me in' census (2005–2010) of patients and service users in mental health and learning disability hospitals demonstrated well the differences in occupancy rates between minority groups. Chinese people had the lowest occupancy ratios (substantially below average), Black British the highest (much above average). Indian were lower than average, White British just below the mean, and other groups were progressively more likely to be detained in the order of Pakistani and Bangladeshi, Mixed groups, Black Caribbean, Black African and highest were Black British (mainly young Black people) (CQC, 2011). There was no simple Black–White distinction, which suggests the reasons are complex.

However, this misses a critical point about values. The values espoused by Black people about mental health care have been shaped over many years. There is a genuine fear of mental health services given the number of Black African-Caribbean people who have died during control and restraint procedures (e.g. the David 'Rocky' Bennett Inquiry report, 2003); a belief that they will not be treated well in hospital (and there are striking figures about such things as time-out); and a lack of confidence that there will be treatments available that meet their needs (see, for example, Department of Health, 2005). Developing a genuinely values-based service will mean taking these concerns seriously and commissioning care that reflects a true understanding about the community served. That may have a range of implications, such as more Black or minority ethnic staff; focus groups of Black patients; faith-based groups; or Black advocacy arrangements.

Working with minority groups demands patience and a commitment to ensuring that the research benefits the group directly, not the researcher or the funding body. This can be achieved by working with communities in new and exacting ways. Training volunteer researchers within communities; obtaining research funding that is free of bias and control; working in those communities with staff who have a similar ethnicity, or gender, or language. One project undertook research into the reasons that south Asian heritage mothers did not use statutory services in Blackburn, and utilised two members of staff, both Muslim women who spoke Urdu fluently. Another project with the gay and lesbian community in Manchester recognised the strongly held values of equality and acceptance, recognition and redistribution, which underwrote the project. Both projects respected the nature of the group and their values as critical to success.

Conclusion: engagement and recognition

Recognition is an important value in commissioning (Fraser and Honneth, 2003). Recognising ethnicity, gender, or faith places a responsibility on the commissioner to redistribute resources to meet their needs in proportion to their recognised importance. That may mean existing services being cut or curtailed, with the attendant opposition that will inevitably occur. That is better than perpetuating a system that is at once unfair and likely to (re-)create further inequality. By listening to the group or community it will be possible, slowly at first and then with increasing speed and emphasis, to develop a portfolio of services that represent a values-based reflection of the needs of the whole community.

Engaging all sections of the community, especially minority groups, is an essential characteristic of values-based practice. How this is done will depend on the nature of the group and the questions to be asked. By working with all cultures and shades of opinion commissioners will be able to balance competing demands more reasonably and address the discriminations felt and expressed by minority communities.

The 'new' public health

The public health function has a wide-ranging overview of health, well-being and social care, although for almost 40 years until recently it was seen as a 'health', that is an NHS, function. Older people may remember the Medical Officer of Health (MoH), a local government post that provided a model which will be more or less recreated in a new form as a result of the government's changes. Public health has been given relatively little credit over the years, certainly not by the general population who have little understanding of its role, for the important part it plays in society, alongside environmental health services provided by local authorities. Now that the public health function is to move to local government there is scope for a greater visibility in demonstrating its value to the community, although conversely less visibility as an NHS function.

For many years, public health has undertaken broadly four separate tasks for health authorities, latterly, PCTs, and now local authorities. It has tackled prevention and health promotion, often in conjunction with health-promotion teams; it has dealt with communicable disease control, notably keeping an eye on epidemics and outbreaks of cryptosporidium and other micro-organisms, and in organising or promoting vaccination programmes; it has tackled health inequalities and equity gaps in health and social care, not least in working with local government in the Spearhead group and similar initiatives; and it has undertaken a large number of reviews of strategic needs as part of support to health authority and PCT boards on priority setting and resource allocation.

Public health has been given new responsibilities and will now move into local government to support Health and Well-being Boards and a new agenda tackling health and social inequalities, based in large measure on the Marmot Review that placed an emphasis on social determinants of health (Marmot Review, 2010). The revised public health processes will include equity gap analysis, challenging health inequalities, and recognising the importance of the (mental) health and well-being agenda. The latter especially will provide a major opportunity to deal with the worst aspects of health and social care, and to develop priority-setting proposals to ensure that the worst examples of socially constructed illness are rooted out.

This latter challenge is one that will demand sophisticated political skills. The money available is tight at a time when the NHS is expected to find up to £20 billion in savings for re-investment, and local authority services are being cut by up to 30% overall, in some cases by much more. For example, Haringey youth budget has been cut by 75% in 2011–12 (http://www.haringey.gov.uk/council_guide_2011–12.pdf); Bolton exemplified 45% cuts in expenditure in 2011 during the cost-cutting exercise (http://menmedia.co.uk/manchestereveningnews/news/s/1406168_1500_jobs_face_axe_in_bolton_council_cuts_worth_60m).

This is time for careful but assertive analysis of the well-being interventions with a structured set of proposals to achieve changes to service profiles that meet the QIPP agenda.

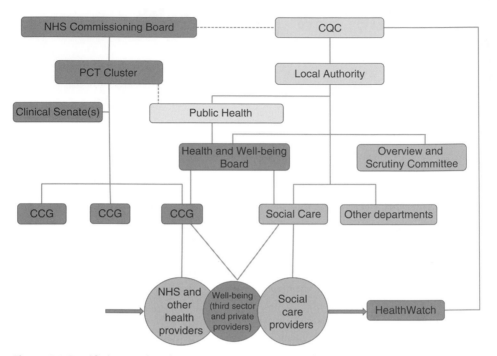

Figure 6.1 Simplified approach to the recent government proposals for the NHS and social care.

As Andrew Lansley said on 2 July 2010: 'All those who work on the frontline should be thinking carefully, and imaginatively, about how we can do things differently. The QIPP process is a home for this in the NHS and the way that we can implement the best and brightest ideas across the service.' And as David Cameron said: 'Don't hold back – be innovative, be radical, challenge the way things are done' (Taylor, 2011).

Figure 6.1 shows a stylised version of the likely structural features of the new arrangements. Those elements in dark grey are all new; those in light grey are elements that remain from before; and the public health component is the only one that has changed, moved from PCTs to local authorities, but retaining a role in both health and local authority management.

The important points to note are that (1) the PCT clusters are likely to remain after the reforms are completed, (2) the CCGs will have a real say but will not have the autonomy that GPCCs thought they would have, and (3) the various parties will be responsible separately and together for health, well-being and social care. In many cases CCGs will be locked into a relationship with Health and Well-being Boards, especially where there is coterminosity between health and local government. The role of Monitor is discussed in Chapter 9 as it plays relatively little part in the considerations of public health.

NICE produces independent evidence-based public health guidance on ways of improving health and well-being for local authorities, education, voluntary organisations and community groups as well as the NHS. As the lead responsibility for public health moves to local government, work with local authorities to explore how well-evidenced and cost-effective public health activities can be used to improve local services and accountability to local communities.

Figure 6.2 is intended to capture two cyclical programmes: the outer circle is the health and well-being commissioning programme and the inner circle is the public health

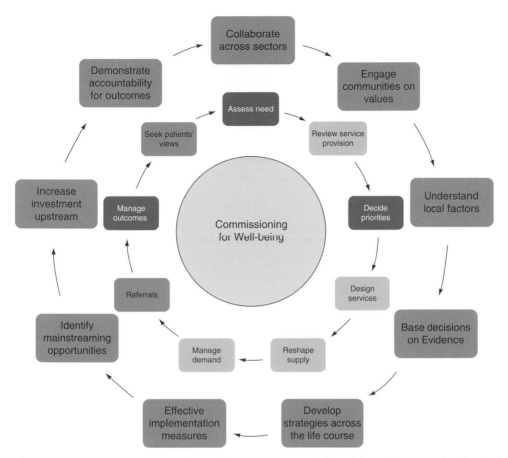

Figure 6.2 The outer circle is the Canadian Model Commissioning Cycle for Well-being. The inner circle is the APHO cycle for commissioning. The darker segments show the present focus of public health; the four light grey segments show some involvement of public health.

programme. The critical difference is in relation to priorities. In the outer circle we assume a simple model of evidence-based priorities. This is because the evidence for prevention and health promotion is good in some areas, relatively poor in some, and not robust in others. Thus the priorities essentially choose themselves on the basis of the evidence alone. In the inner circle we have a more traditional, managerial evidence-based programme. Public health by its own admission is most associated with assessing need, deciding priorities and managing outcomes (APHO website). By factoring into the public health domain the important features of the outer circle (such as explicitly determining values, life-course programmes and upstream interventions) it will be possible to achieve a more powerful and genuinely holistic programme, as described in the first government priority above.

Fair society, healthy lives

Fair society, healthy lives: The Marmot Review report was published in February 2010 (Marmot Review, 2010; www.marmotreview.org). The report has been influential not only in the UK, but also internationally. For example, the World Health Organisation established a Commission on the Social Determinants of Health between 2005 and 2008 to support countries and global health partners address the social factors leading to ill health and inequities, and this has led to a programme to tackle equity gaps in health care. The Marmot Review covered a number of important matters in relation to health inequalities and discussed, among other things, (a) the importance of focusing on social determinants of health, and (b) using the notion of proportionate universalism to devise a strategy to combat inequalities.

Marmot describes the way that social determinants play a major role in the development of disease, and suggests that a programme to tackle these issues should create an enabling society to maximise individual and community potential, and ensure that social justice, health and sustainability are at the heart of policy initiatives. The six areas for action in England are: giving every child the best start in life, enabling everyone to have control over their lives, creating fair employment and good work for all, ensuring a healthy standard of living for all, creating and developing healthy and sustainable places and communities, and strengthening the role and impact of prevention of illness. This is reflected in the World Health Organisation programme on social determinants of health, within which Sir Michael Marmot played a major role.

Many practitioners have found helpful Marmot's emphasis on 'proportionate universalism', or as at least one Foundation Trust (FT) has proposed, 'progressive universalism', in the way we target populations at risk. Proportionate universalism is a way of describing the balance that must be struck between general interventions that do not discriminate between recipients and those that are risk-targeted at specific groups. For example, parenting skills have been identified as a critical ingredient in the development of good social skills in children: we know that poor upbringing (especially if mothers suffer from post-natal depression) can be a risk factor for poor attainment and lack of self-esteem during teenage years. Proportionate universalism maintains that all parents should be given opportunities for help and parenting support; and some parents that have either demonstrated a risk profile or who are shown to have some deprivation that makes them eligible will be offered increasingly expensive interventions to assist with their parenting skills.

Figure 6.3 shows what this means for universal parenting support and the increasingly targeted programmes made available as assessed risk increases. In fact, these matters had been the driver for the New Horizons programme at the DH, and a programme to combat health and social inequalities.

Although the main thrust of the Spearhead group of Local Authorities inequalities programme has been completed, it is more than likely that the new public health arrangements within local authorities will pick this up and form it into the basis of a composite Clinical Commissioning Group–Health and Well-being Board (H&WB) programme. Indeed, the original Spearhead programme has not gone away, as we can see from the extensive data sets available to public health practitioners. There is no doubt, however, that the initial drive has faded even though the task has not been completed.

A revised programme that draws on Marmot, Wanless, health inequalities commissioning (based on the Institute for Innovation and Improvement, 3Is) strategy, together with local and national public health is essential. We can see the clash of values informing the debate. While local authorities have not made as much progress as was hoped, the need to retain and expand the programme is essential. Placing a premium on health inequalities and addressing the social determinants that relate to poorer health is a value that is well worth preserving. The cost is high, however, and it will be essential for public health practitioners to

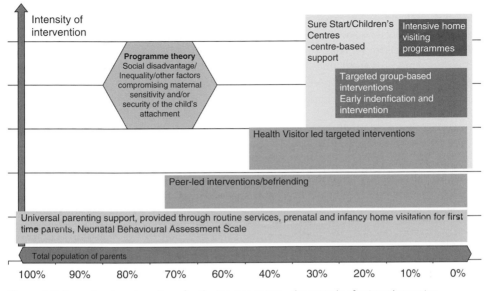

Figure 6.3 Proportionate universalism after the Marmot review – the example of universal parenting.

make a strong case for investment in prevention and health promotion at a time of hospital closures and reductions in the availability of medicines and other treatments.

We might say, similarly, that having effective immunisation programmes is an essential component of any health system. In this case there is no argument about its effectiveness, although ensuring programme viability against those who would undermine herd immunity requires constant vigilance. (See, for example, the case of the MMR triple vaccine described below and available at: http://news.bbc.co.uk/onthisday/hi/dates/stories/january/22/newsid_2506000/2506679.stm.) Smoking and heart attack is another well-proven link which has been amenable to interventions to stop smoking. In this case, however, it has not worked as well as some would have liked and demands further efforts (note the implications for the Wanless review: see Chapter 4).

Some public health initiatives impact on the whole community. Clean water, good air quality, speed restrictions in towns and near schools, and so on, all have wide benefits. On the other hand, there are those where the proportionate universalist argument needs to be considered carefully. Interventions to stop obesity have a universal appeal, but it is only those over a body mass index (BMI) of 25 (overweight) or perhaps 30 (obese) that will benefit dramatically if they follow the advice given; while fluoridation, for example, may have some possible minor harmful effects (or may not provide any direct benefit). All of these examples testify to the value of public health – ensuring that there is a public-funded programme that offers positive health benefits as well as addressing disease burdens.

The Marmot Review report included some suggested indicators to support monitoring of the overall strategic direction in reducing health inequalities. The London Health Observatory and the Marmot Review team produced baseline figures for some important indicators of the social determinants of health, health outcomes and social inequality that correspond, as closely as is currently possible, to the indicators proposed in 'Fair society, healthy lives'.

As we can see in Figures 6.4 and 6.5, between 1981 and 2007, estimates of life expectancy (LE) and disability-free life expectancy (DFLE) at birth in the UK increased for both males and females; healthy life expectancy (HLE) at birth in the period 1981–2006 also increased for each sex. In 2007 LE for females was 81.7 years compared with 77.4 years for males, although the difference has narrowed since 1981. The difference between estimates of LE and HLE/DFLE can be regarded as the number of years a person can expect to live in poor general health or with a limiting persistent illness or disability. In 2007, DFLE at birth was 64.6 years

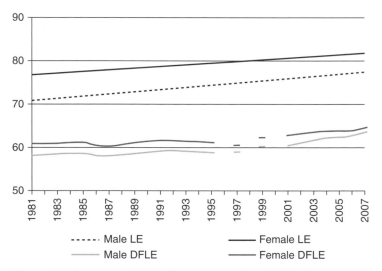

Figure 6.4 Life expectancy, healthy life expectancy and EU – healthy life expectancy at birth, Great Britain 1981–2006 (by permission of the ONS; under the Open Government Licence v.1.0).

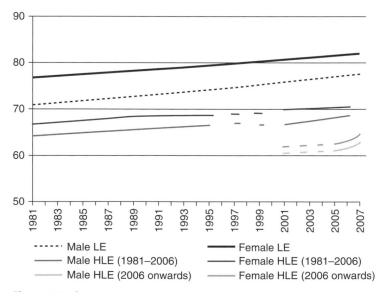

Figure 6.5 Life expectancy and healthy life expectancy for males and females in Great Britain at birth, 1981–2007 (by permission of the ONS; under the Open Government Licence v.1.0).

for females compared with 63.7 years for males. In 1981, males at birth could expect to spend 12.8 years of their life with a limiting persistent illness or disability, compared with 13.7 years in 2007. For females, these figures were 16.0 and 17.1 years, respectively (ONS, 2011).

The infant mortality (IM) target was intended to reduce by at least 10% the gap in mortality between the routine and manual occupation group and the population as a whole. The LE target was intended to reduce by at least 10% by 2010 the gap between the areas with the worst health and deprivation indicators (the 'Spearhead' group – approximately a fifth of all areas) and England as a whole (relative to a 1995–97 baseline). The Spearhead Group of 70 Local Authority (single-tier and district council) areas (which following the NHS reconfiguration overlap with 62 PCTs) are in the bottom fifth nationally for three or more of the following five factors:

- male life expectancy at birth;
- female life expectancy at birth;
- cancer mortality rate in under 75s;
- cardiovascular disease mortality rate in under 75s; or
- Index of Multiple Deprivation 2004 (Local Authority Summary) average score.

Achievement of these target figures across all PCT footprints was expected to deliver required progress against the national targets for overall LE and inequalities in LE, given specified assumptions about England average performance. The indicative figures for the Spearhead elements also incorporated a degree of 'stretch', to allow for the possibility that the England average may exceed expected performance, and to ensure that the gap between Spearhead areas and the England average still decreases sufficiently if an England 'overachievement' actually occurred. Nationally, the data have shown substantial improvements in LE, including those in disadvantaged groups and areas, compared with the baseline periods; however, the gap between male and female LE has increased.

Health-related behaviour in the Spearhead areas has shown paradoxical and contrary changes. For example, while smoking appears to have fallen in both affluent and deprived groups, the ratio between the two groups has increased from 132% to 169%, suggesting that the gap has not narrowed. Conversely, obesity has increased in both affluent and deprived communities, although by somewhat less in the deprived community, thus narrowing the gap. A similar pattern was found in the non-Spearhead areas. After smoking, the most marked difference between affluent and deprived communities was the prevalence of Type II diabetes, where the gap had narrowed from 101% in 2002 to 77% in 2009 (Hippisley-Cox, 2009).

Some progress has been made, but not sufficient to be satisfied that the strategy is working well. We can see from Figures 6.6 and 6.7 the challenge, and the opportunity in relation to life expectancy. An online tool is now available for local authorities to check their own data on four interventions. These are:

- smoking cessation;
- interventions to reduce infant mortality;
- treatment with anti-hypertensive drugs; and
- treatment with statins.

By setting out the problem in this way, it is evident just how much needs to be done to improve LE, and where we should place our resources. Improving LE for all, but especially

Female life expectancy at birth, inequality gap*
England 1993–200 and target projection for the year '2010'

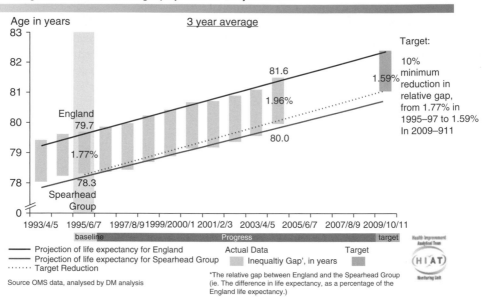

Age in years

3 year average

Target:

10% minimum reduction in relative gap, from 1.77% in 1995–97 to 1.59% In 2009–911

— Projection of life expectancy for England
— Projection of life expectancy for Spearhead Group
······ Target Reduction

Actual Data
Inequaltiy Gap', in years
Target

Source OMS data, analysed by DM analysis

*The relative gap between England and the Spearhead Group (ie. The difference in life expectancy, as a percentage of the England life expectancy.)

The Gap – for females

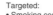

30% All circulatory diseases, 63% of which are Coronary Heart Disease (CHD)

16% All cancers, 75% of which are lung cancer

21% Respiratory diseases, 57% of which are chronic obstructive airways disease

9% Digestive, 44% of which are chronic liver disease and cirrhosis
5% External causes of injury and poisoning, 40% of which are suicide and undertermined death
2% infectious and parasitic diseases
11% Other
6% Deaths under 28 days

Contribution to Life Expectancy Gap in Females
Breakdown by disease, 2003

The Interventions

Targeted:
• Smoking cessation clinics: double capacity in Spearhead areas for years
• Secondary prevention of CVD: additional 15% coverage of effective therapies in Spearhead areas 35–74 yrs
• Primary prevention of CVD in hypertensives under 75 yrs:
    40% coverage antihypertensives statin therapy
• Primary prevention of CVD in hypertensives 75 yrs +:
    40% coverage antihypertensives statin therapy
• Other' including:
    Early detection of cancer
    Respiratory diseases
    Alcohol related diseases
    Infant mortality   *locally determined

Universalist:
• Smoking reduction in clinics – as at present
• Secondary prevention of CVD: 75% coverage of 35–74 yrs
• Primary prevention of CVD in hyptensives under 75 yrs:
    20% coverage antihypertensive statin therapy

The Impact – for females

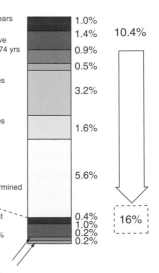

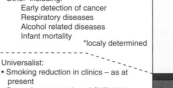

1.0%
1.4%   10.4%
0.9%
0.5%

3.2%

1.6%

5.6%

0.4%
1.0%   16%
0.2%
0.2%

Figure 6.6 Spearhead group illustrations showing the extent of difference in life expectancy and the way the gap is made up for females (by permission of the Department of Health; under the Open Government Licence v.1.0).

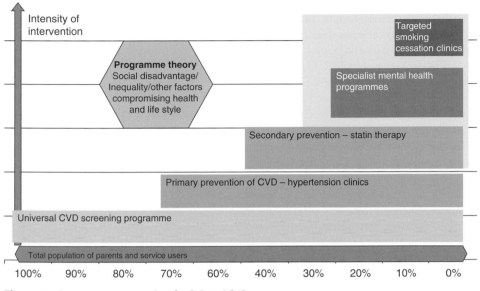

Figure 6.7 Proportionate universalism for CVD and CHD.

those whose LE is lower as a result of deprivation, is an important value. Although Figure 6.6 is for 2002–2004, and thus rather out of date, it demonstrates the relevance of the programme.

Similar graphs are available for males and females. For female LE the 'gap' between the least-deprived and the most-deprived households is made up of 30% all circulatory diseases, 16% all cancers, 21% respiratory diseases, 9% digestive disorders, and 24% other causes. On the right-hand side of the diagram we can see the proposed 'solutions': targeted smoking cessation, CVD and CHD programmes with an emphasis on hypertension and statin therapy. We might create a diagram, similar to that shown earlier, showing the way CVD risk can be dealt with. A universal CVD screening programme leads onto more targeted interventions for those at heightened risk.

The important point to note is the way values are inter-related. Two sets of values matter. The first set of values contains those of public health itself – those values directed to resolving health inequalities demonstrates a genuine and valid attempt to make amends for 'prior discriminations', patients ignored or abandoned by the health and social care system, poor quality care, and little support or assistance for those living in deprivation. In the second set are those values held by the patients and service users themselves (Diagrams 17 and 18). What do these graphs tell us about those values, and the way in which we must work with patients to tackle these problems? If we simply apply medical or managerial paternalism we will not make much headway with those whom we are trying to help. Only by engaging the groups of like service users, or similar communities, in a values-based approach will it be possible to make real and sustained progress.

Marmot indicators

The Marmot Review report included some suggested indicators to support monitoring of the overall strategic direction in reducing health inequalities. The London Health Observatory and the Marmot Review Team have produced baseline figures for some key indicators of the social determinants of health, health outcomes and social inequality that correspond, as closely as is currently possible, to the indicators proposed in 'Fair society, healthy lives' (http://www.lho.org.uk/lho_topics/national_lead_areas/Marmot/MarmotIndicators.aspx).

Most of the Marmot indicators reflect disparities in LE, with others picking up the six key recommendations of the review.[1] While these are valuable for public health within local authorities, the APHO also issued in 2011 a range of new small area (MSOA)[2] indicators to support public health and social care in undertaking JSNA (http://www.apho.org.uk/RESOURCE/VIEW.ASPX?RID=87735).

The indicators include population estimates, mortality, hospitalisation, lifestyle and socio-economic data (2011). A thorough understanding of an area requires 'information about the component parts of the area at the smallest level consistent with reliability, robustness, completeness, and confidentiality' (APHO, 2011). Although the motivating factor was JSNA, the data sets produced will be useful across a range of health-profiling and needs-assessment activities.

However, the indicators quite understandably do not recognise explicitly the values of groups within the population. The data sets are intended to cover a range of issues, focused on underlying determinants of health and conditions which account for substantial numbers of preventable diseases and deaths. They have been divided into domains covering different aspects of health needs:

- population/demography,
- socio-economic indicators,
- lifestyle/behaviour,
- mortality/life expectancy, and
- hospitalisation/service utilisation.

---

[1] The indicators are:

- male LE,
- female LE,
- slope index of inequality (SII) for male LE,
- SII for female LE,
- SII for male DFLE,
- SII for female DFLE,
- children achieving a good level of development at age 5,
- young people who are not in education, employment or training (NEET),
- people in households in receipt of means-tested benefits, and SII for people in households in receipt of means-tested benefits.

[2] The smallest geographical area used is the Middle Level Super Output Area (MSOA), chosen because they are well established, durable, small enough to produce a range of results for almost every Local Authority (LA)/Unitary Authority (UA) and sufficiently large for the results to be reliable. MSOAs have an average population of 7200 people, which generally produces sufficient numbers of cases to prevent disclosure of information about identifiable individuals, and thus there are relatively few indicators suppressed.

It is intended that the data set will be updated annually. However, a separate project is reviewing the content and the previously published APHO core data set for JSNA, so it is likely that the current content of the data sets will be rationalised, and extended to include projections and comparisons of observed and expected results. To be useful in commissioning, however, will require a focus on the values of the population or communities covered. Involving public health practitioners with commissioning staff in understanding the values of the communities served will further enhance the programme to tackle health inequalities.

The 'new' public health

The White Paper, 'Healthy lives, healthy people: Our strategy for public health in England', offers a real challenge to local authorities (Department of Health, 2011a). From April 2013 upper tier and unitary authorities will take the public health functions. Four key changes are proposed.

- Local authorities will have new responsibilities for public health, with new opportunities for community engagement and 'holistic' solutions to health and well-being with a form of 'total place' commissioning.
- A new, integrated public health service will support local action and especially a focus on outcomes.
- Public health will be a 'core part of business' in central government.
- There is a commitment to reduce health inequalities and support for the Marmot review to address the 'wider' determinants.

The vision for the system is – must be – shaped by a set of values. It will be expected to be responsive to and 'owned' by the communities to which it is responsible; funded from ring-fenced resources with incentives for improvement; professionally led and focused on evidence; resilient about current and future threats to health. Once more, we can see that the values of the community are not explicitly stated, although the question of how the public health programme is 'owned' by the communities served is left open to interpretation. The whole system will be 'focussed around achieving positive health outcomes for the population, rather than on process targets . . .' (Department of Health, 2011a, p. 10).

Local authorities will be required to deliver or commission public health services where services need to be provided universally, the Secretary of State is under a legal duty (but is likely to delegate the responsibility), and that certain steps that are 'critical to the running of public health' will be taken (Department of Health, 2011a, p. 12). By and large, this means appropriate access to sexual health services, health protection, child health programmes, Health Check programmes, and ensuring that NHS commissioners receive public health advice. Whether public health will have a real role in working with CCGs to tackle priority-setting, resource allocation and rationing decisions is unclear, as is their role with values rather than evidence. It suggests that emphasising values is essential as this new system beds down.

Some things will continue, nonetheless. Ensuring herd immunity is an important goal of public health. Promoting immunisation programmes and working with GPs, school nurses and occupational health programmes will remain and become ever more necessary with the expansion of international travel and increased migration. New diseases and adaptation by existing ones will need careful monitoring. From a values-based perspective we can say two things: first that 'public health' is a value that we should cherish – in other words, having a powerful public health programme that is well-funded and appropriately organised; and second that we must be alert to potential changes that undermine the programme, whether as a result of political interference, organisational change, or professional differences.

The recent debate on implications of the triple vaccine (measles, mumps and rubella, MMR) (McGreevy, 2005) was caused by a paper in the *Lancet* (Wakefield *et al.*, 1998).[3] This was reported widely by the media and generated alarm in parents of young children, and contributed to their refusal to let their children have the triple vaccine. Two things were evident from the public debate: first, many people were not able adequately or were disinclined to consider the science presented carefully by doctors once it was clear that the Wakefield paper was wrong (Madsen *et al.*, 2002); and second, parents did not accept as a values imperative, even after the refutation of Wakefield's paper, the idea and importance of herd immunity. This suggests, as the debate on the future of the NHS indicates, that we have as a society forgotten the important reasons why we do some things that were established many years ago. Public health may need to develop a forceful public education programme to reinforce the requisite good surveillance systems and to put resources into ensuring robust organisations and rapid reaction to threat.

Community, connectedness and climate change

Public health has an enormously important job to do over the next few years. Adopting the 'connectedness' shown in Figure 6.8, it may be possible to effect a transformation in the way that communities and local government tackle health and well-being (see New Horizons: Department of Health, 2009). Indeed, New Horizons was before its time in promoting resilience and connectedness as shown in Figure 6.8.

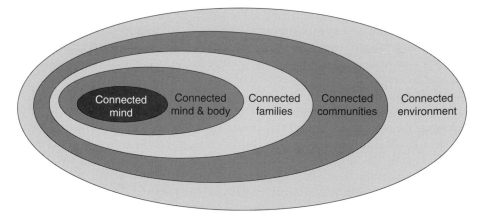

Figure 6.8 Connected ecosystem of health and social systems (*Source*: Dr Jo Nurse, New Horizons Programme, 2008, Department of Health).

---

[3] Following investigation initially by the Sunday Times and then later by the General Medical Council, the author was found to be guilty of serious professional misconduct and struck off the medical register. However, the scare that the publication of the 1998 paper created took 10 years to die down, despite a partial retraction by the Lancet in 2004, followed by a full retraction in 2010.

Although not explicitly stated, the New Horizons programme, while ostensibly concerned with population (positive) mental health, anticipated future discussion on a range of challenges to public health, including the empowerment of communities, the importance of green solutions to many problems, and notably climate change and global warming (see McKibben, 2010). Public health will have to take the brunt of the responsibility for the implications of tackling health inequalities, cuts to services, and protecting the health of the population. To this is now added a pressure from the health-related aspects of climate change (such as changing patterns of disease vectors). Climate change poses a severe problem for public health from the difficulties associated with sudden floods and storm damage to the mental health implications of acute exacerbations of the weather. Present establishment values emphasise economic growth while undertaking some background work on differing energy alternatives, but they do not give sufficient weight to the health implications of global warming. Population anxieties will become ever more prevalent as climate change implicated events become ever more frequent.

The values of communities will eventually take over from the values of those in power, but, sadly, as one health economist was fond of saying, 'it's always too soon until, suddenly, it's too late.' If public health is to reflect the real pressures on health and health services, there will need to be an authoritative programme not just to tackle health inequalities, important as that is given that people living in deprived communities are likely to be hit hardest by the effects of climate change, but also to tackle the increasingly obvious implications of climate change itself. Heatstroke, vector-borne diseases and acute anxiety are just a few of the likely effects that will increase, possibly quite quickly over the next 5–10 years. Commissioning health and social care must reflect these changes, but has not done so to date.

Conclusion

Public health has an enormously important role to play, now and in future. For it to do so requires a values-based approach that engages all service users to understand what is acceptable to the service users targeted, especially in tackling ingrained and persistent health inequalities. The opportunity afforded by the proposed move to local authorities offers the chance to challenge all aspects of lifestyle choices from a values-based perspective.

Integrative commissioning for health and social care

Integrated or joint commissioning

Integrative commissioning is the terminology adopted for commissioning jointly from health and social care agencies and from the third sector as well as from other agencies, such as the Education Department of the local authority or the Police or Probation Service. In this chapter we will consider the way that local authorities, health agencies, the third sector and other agencies can and have worked together to commission a range of services that link together for the purposes of achieving a good mix of services. Whether we have a short-term collage of services or a longer-term integrated provision is less important than the agreement to develop, plan, and commission together.

The chapter considers the way that we obtain information about 'need' and how that relates to the 'values' of the people whose needs we have ascertained. This will be complemented by discussions about:

- needs-based commissioning – of health and social care together with JSNA;
- integrated commissioning – the joint and agreed approach that develops from V-BP and E-BM;
- health economic and epidemiological models;
- culturally relevant assessment and diagnosis – of disease and illness; and
- choice and personalisation.

Integrative commissioning builds on JSNA to develop a set of needs and aspirations, strengths and opportunities. The JSNA is a valuable resource, but is also rather overwhelming in its scope. Many local authorities have now finalised their first cut JSNA and they make interesting reading. By and large, the opportunity has been taken to describe the 'facts' of needs assessment without the 'values' that run alongside. Setting out the needs in this way, especially from a public health perspective, provides a good template for action. The problem then becomes, 'what action?' In social services (child and families, and adult) the most significant actions will be those that deal with the reduction in funding and the development of new market ideologies. In Chapter 9 we will see the extent to which the market can address the changes that are needed.

Integrative commissioning – the joint and agreed approach that develops from V-BP and E-BM – is the way that integrated commissioning draws on and shapes the values base and the evidence base both naturally and scientifically. Integrated commissioning goes beyond a simple distinction of old-style commissioning to a new and detailed understanding of the

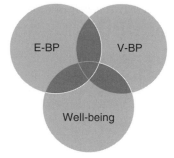

Figure 7.1 Evidence, Values and Well-being inter-relate.

different commissioning tasks and the key elements of that task. The framework is one that brings together health care commissioning, social care arrangements and other bodies to try to devise a formula that is at once agreeable but is also distinct.

V-BP and E-BM are two parts of a whole. This can be illustrated by Figure 7.1. The left-hand circle shows E-BP and the right-hand circle V-BP: the right-hand circle shows how the changes will develop; the left-hand circle the way the changes will work. The 'well-being' section holds the 'common' elements, those that are largely tied to the well-being agenda that local authorities will manage in collaboration.

Personalisation requires a focus on the individual as the person whose support and life care is determined by the two main commissioners – health and medicine on the one hand, social care and life opportunities on the other. In some cases the individual will require medical care only – say, diabetes care supported by a diabetes primary care team; in other cases only social care will be needed, without any other medium- or longer-term care – say, residential care. In other cases, the individual will require the support of both: for a neurological disorder, a personalised budget for neurological support, supplied by the GP, and a day care support worker to deal with the ever-present physical inability to dress and manage activities of daily living (ADL). In this case the opportunity to develop a joint health and social care budget is powerful, bringing together the health and social care elements.

The third element is well-being, including prevention and health promotion. If we take the last of our examples we can see that medical treatment and residential care is probably insufficient for the person to have a 'good' life. Almost certainly a neurological disorder will be disabling to a degree, and the person's inability to dress and manage ADL tasks will compound the effects of that disorder. The well-being element will be invaluable to the person's positive mental health. This could include additional support in the workplace if relevant or to take exercise and visit relatives; or support to take a voluntary post dealing with green spaces development.

Integrative commissioning is the term used to describe the agreement between health and social care agencies to create together a self-made commissioning process between the GP (and the primary care team) and the social care team, with others engaged as necessary. The reason this has not happened so far is a reluctance on the part of GPs and social care staff to give up what they both see as their territory, to lose power and control. Yet if values-based commissioning is to mean anything it demands that power and control is shared as widely as possible. There will be those professional staff who will not under any circumstances allow this to happen. This is strange when what we are concerned about is those times when either the values of the service user are at odds with the professional commissioners, or the clinician does not have a good answer to the patient's needs. In these cases surely it is better, even on a 'protect my back' basis, to share the responsibility with the patient or service user.

There will also be the need to identify one or more commissioners as those who have the responsibility for negotiating an agreement with providers and agreeing the spend. Commissioning for 'personalisation' and 'person-centred care' requires that commissioning staff recognise and understand this and accept that person-centredness requires a joint and integrative process that values the service user as a person with rights and responsibilities entitled to be engaged fully and cooperatively in the practice of deciding on the best care for her and her colleagues.

Integrated commissioning is, 'a single system of needs determination and service commissioning ... to improve the quality and appropriateness of services and support received by users ... and ... service user expectations' (Thistlethwaite, 2011). Conversely, Joint Commissioning is a 'process in which two or more organisations act together to coordinate the commissioning of services, taking joint responsibility for the translation of strategy into action'. On the other hand, integrated commissioning takes a wider role and urges 'joint health and social care ... to encompass a wider range of partners with the aim of addressing the needs of individuals and communities in a holistic way', and goes on to specify Local Strategic Partnerships as one of a number of bodies that could be used (Carson *et al.*, 2010). *Integrative* commissioning seeks to bring these together, to recognise that 'integrative' is a process, an on-going system of finding support and guidance, of working with service users and commissioners in a unified whole.

Integrative commissioning implies a wider responsibility to ensure that all agencies are engaged and empowered. If one of our 'values' is that 'integration is good', it is essential we consider carefully what we mean. However, do we mean integration, or integrative? Ensuring that all agencies work closely together, indeed are interwoven in their pursuit of high-quality care, is not the same as saying that we want wholesale 'integration'. Many readers will know of Leutz's five (now six) laws of Integration (Leutz, 1999, 2005) which bear repeating here:

Law 1: *You can integrate some of the services all of the time, all of the services some of the time, but you can't integrate all of the services all of the time*. Integrating services, or more appropriately commissioning of services, should be considered carefully. Where are the natural boundaries between agencies or functions? By trying to integrate everything, in practice we end up by fragmenting the new arrangement. Perhaps a better way to tackle integration is to identify those services that target those individuals or families with complex needs or complex solutions. Will integration of commissioning (perhaps between CCGs and Health and Well-being Boards) achieve the end of integrating services; and what do we mean by integration. Do we mean not 'seamless' but closely stitched seams? Or do we mean *true* integration in one organisation?

Law 2: *Integration costs before it pays*. Integration can lead to initial double running costs. 'Pump priming' needs to be considered and allowed for, and the overall costs assessed before embarking on potentially unnecessary integration processes. Again it is worth asking: what will integration achieve? Will it achieve improvements in care?

Law 3: *Your integration is my fragmentation*. This may explain why many people resist integration – integrating, say, primary care with local government social care will create a fissure or obstruction between primary care and acute in-patient care. It will be essential to consider what may be lost through integration as to what is likely to be gained.

Law 4: *You can't integrate a square peg into a round hole.* Of course, this is contentious. Some policy positions may remain permanent challenges. However, from a V-BP perspective there may be differing values sets that can be accommodated by 'agreeing to disagree' ('dissensus') on one or two values while recognising that others are simply different ways of saying the same thing. Local government charge for many services, the health service does not, and this has been used as an excuse over the years for inaction. However, recognising where the service user and the professional staff can agree rather than where they might disagree suggests a small number of difficulties that can then be readily mitigated.

Law 5: *The person who integrates calls the tune.* 'Whilst this may appear to be a comment on relative organisational and professional power, it is not. The argument instead is for integration to be the result of designs by those who use the services, rather than professionals – a call for rapid moves towards meeting the personalisation agenda' (Walker, 2008). By turning the integration agenda on its head and empowering patients and service users to encourage, indeed force, professionals to integrate their services, we will achieve a much faster transformation of health and social care.

Law 6: *All integration is local.* Local leadership is essential to implementation and innovative outcomes. We will see in Chapter 10 the way that leadership can affect the changes in local leadership that are needed.

Whole systems

The QIPP 'Right Care' workstream is focused on enabling clinicians and commissioners to deliver the best value from health resources as the NHS moves through the current transition programme. This will be achieved by supporting healthcare organisations to develop sustainable systems and pathways of care and a focus on reducing unwarranted variation in clinical practice. The methods used to support these processes include a strong focus on programme budgeting as well as detailed analysis using spend and outcomes tools. In Chapter 7 we will see the way that programme budgeting and marginal analysis (PBMA) offers a way to identify those programmes that are expensive in comparison to other areas. It allows us to ask questions and to derive answers that we then test locally.

'Right Care' is focused on increasing value' in three ways.

- Ensuring resources are allocated in the best possible way by commissioners.
- Doing the right things. This means shifting spend from lower-value areas to higher-value areas and ensuring that patients will continue to receive best 'value' care (note that 'value' here is used in the sense of 'value for money').
- Helping the individual patient or service user to make a decision that is right for their values (and note, here it is used as we have been using the term 'values').

The programme offers the opportunity to focus on value (as value for money, VFM) and on values. The first question that comes to mind is: can VFM or monetary value equate in any way to 'values of values-based practice'? To what extent can V-BP be hijacked to support a VFM agenda without being corrupted internally? Can VFM be bound up with V-BP such that achieving VFM is morally and practically acceptable? Consequently, if Right Care works as it should, it will bring *values* as well as *value* centre stage.

A whole-systems approach is a pre-requisite to effective commissioning. Using stocks and flows models it is possible to show how whole systems in modelling and design of services can save significant resources.[1] One of the most important aspects of health care development over the transition period has actually been the lack of whole-systems thinking, despite an insistence on place-based budgets. It will not be possible to achieve the best and most cost-effective service if we think in narrow vertical 'silos' and do not link together all services and supports in a community and for an individual: health and social care and other departments of local authorities (education, transport, housing, and so on) with the police, probation and the prison service.

'Strategies to achieve these outcomes must be based on the identification and support of all community assets, [which] includes public services, but goes much further to include citizens, families and the full range of community resources' (The Centre for Welfare Reform, accessed 19 August 2011). As one commentator has suggested, total place requires 'total commissioning', and a 'joined up view of the customer and their needs. It is about identifying, analysing and managing demand, prioritising the demand that needs to be satisfied and then selecting the most efficient and cost effective means of delivery. This means achieving a fundamental separation between demand and delivery management' (Cherrett, 2010).

However, whole systems are more than 'total place'. An emphasis on whole systems recognises that health and social care systems are intimately inter-related. Primary care, in-patient acute provision, community health and social services, residential and nursing home care, and third-sector support, are all part of an integrated arrangement. Making a change in one component will affect all the others; investing resources in hospital beds without considering the impact on residential or intermediate care may cause more problems than it solves. Partnership is important. The White Paper, 'Creating Strong, Safe and Prosperous Communities' (DCLG, 2008) offered guidance to local authorities and their partners on the operation of the Local Government and Public Involvement in Health Act 2007, and covered Local Strategic Partnerships, Sustainable Community Strategies, the new duty to involve, Local Area Agreements, the revised 'best-value' regime and commissioning.

Proposals for the transformation of health and social care are based on local authority's Health and Well-being Boards and CCGs working closely together to identify local needs through the joint production of a strategic needs assessment, and to establish local priorities in association with a range of organisations, including the third sector, social enterprises and cooperatives. The government's statement on public health, Healthy lives, healthy people (Department of Health, 2011d), 'emphasised the focus on communities as the drivers of public health priorities, rather than centralised targets, ... with priorities set by everyone within a community, not just those who currently use health or social care services' (http://www.yhsccommissioning.org.uk/index.php?pageNo=554).

Commissioning for 'total place' has been taken forward with the advent of 16 Community Budget Pilots that were announced in the 2010 Comprehensive Spending Review. The pilots will pool various elements of government funding into a single 'local bank account' for tackling social problems around families with complex needs. The pool will give the pilots local discretion and accountability with 'direct control over local spending in their area free of centrally imposed conditions'. The organisation responsible for the budget could commission

---

[1] The firm *symmetric* has undertaken a large amount of modelling for the Department of Health and contributed to the programmes on commissioning run by the University of Central Lancashire. Their two key conclusions are: (1) that health and social care is a whole system and must be treated as such; and (2) modelling demonstrates the importance of whole systems methodology, using programmes based on stocks and flows.

other local public organisations to deliver some services for families with complex needs, including the possibility of offering an individual social care (and potentially health care) budget (http://www.instituteforgovernment.org.uk/content/170/community-budgets; http://www.centreforwelfarereform.org/innovations/total-place-commissioning.htmlfor).

From the V-BP perspective, this offers opportunities to discuss values with the community and with individual families. For example, a number of projects have found that tackling well-being for dysfunctional families with complex needs requires an outreach arrangement rather than expecting the families to come to a 'clinic' or explicitly professional service (e.g. the four pilot sites for commissioning health and well-being in the North West demonstrated the importance of the third sector and local government 'detached' well-being coordinators). Simply holding a community budget reveals a range of values. These may be a desire to assist families with complex needs in innovative ways; or it may represent a strong philosophy of 'self-help' that may be sponsored by this process. As a minimum it will be necessary to engage in a values-based discussion with all those agencies involved and with families to understand the way in which the resources can be used to best effect.

Patient and service user care pathways

Patient or service user care pathway re-design is one area that has received a lot of attention, but too often using a simple model of linear pathways. Without recognising the interconnectedness of stages in the pathway and the way that patients and service users travel along (and back and forth) on the pathway, it is impossible to design pathways that can be used by 'real' people in the real world. Many providers are using pathways, but admit that they do not provide an easy assimilation of important information. Sometimes a 'pathway' is simply a statement of stages with quality criteria at each stage, sometimes it is a virtual mechanism for envisioning the pathway, but does not provide a 'real' reflection of what happens to the patient. The importance of pathways is in providing a 'glue' that binds the various professional staff to a stylised process of care. A pathway has the key components that can be referenced and referred to, and it has critical elements of information that may be relevant at different times. However, it is not a pathway as we might think of the Pembroke Coast path, going continuously from point A to point B.

Additionally, each stage of the pathway throws up values questions. This may be about waiting times, access levels, quality considerations (e.g. the way I am spoken to), staff availability at each stage, and so on. A pathway does not necessarily suggest linear progression; no patient is likely to traverse the various elements in exactly the same way. However, the pathway provides a structure and template, plus the opportunity to specify different quality criteria at differing nodes.

The way pathways are thought of is as a branching system, as shown in Figure 7.2, with the patient's route seen as a linear progression along a branch of the pathway. The reality is that a pathway is used as template rather than as a fixed description of the route the patient should (or must) take. Patients make a wide variety of demands on the system and it needs to be sufficiently flexible to accommodate those demands. Understanding patient and service-user values will assist commissioners in designing pathways with sufficient stochastic flexibility, that reflect the actual use made rather than the ideal use that commissioners think is appropriate. A pathway may appear fairly straightforward and linear, as in Figure 7.2.

In practice, patients may well use the pathway non-straightforwardly – perhaps by returning home only to come back and be directed to another service. Following a routine

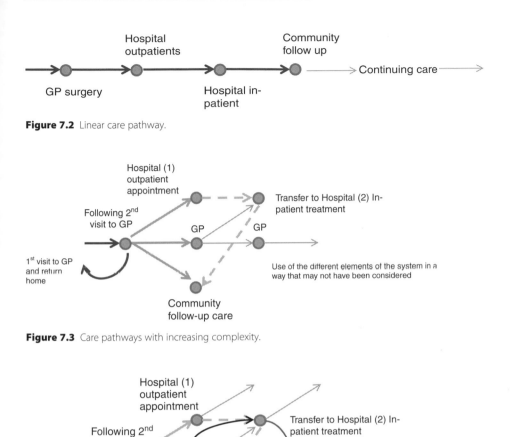

Figure 7.2 Linear care pathway.

Figure 7.3 Care pathways with increasing complexity.

Figure 7.4 Further alternative options.

outpatient appointment the patient is directed to another hospital for treatment, and then is offered follow-up care in the community (Figure 7.3). In practice the route can look even more untidy, especially if we have a range of patients pathways described on it (Figure 7.4).

Care pathways are helpful as ways of describing the values that apply and the outcomes achievable at each stage of the patient's or service-user's journey. However, we should be cautious of using care pathways in a slavish way to describe the specific journey of a patient.

Choice

We have seen that many of the strategies of self-help and personal responsibility for health and social care are predicated on choice. The proposals for community budgets, for example, demand choice by local people, and that will start to put pressure on policy makers to change some of the more problematic policy statements. For example:

- What should be the scope for healthcare free at the point of delivery?
- What is the decent minimum that the state should provide?
- What needs should be met?
- Which 'wants' is it reasonable to accommodate?
- What is the balance between population need and investment to meet individual need?
- What is the reasonable minimum required from social care?

Choice is a double-edged sword. Choice demands pluralism of provision and thus a 'market' in health and social care; choice also places responsibility on the service user to exercise his or her preferences wisely. Choice also implies that personal responsibility is the concomitant of devolved financial support and enhanced personal autonomy. On the other hand, choice demands information and an ability to use the information to a certain degree, and choice places responsibility on the service user to look after herself and seek the best possible care.

Personalisation thus supports taking responsibility for one's own health and doing everything reasonably to stay healthy. That could mean paying for health and well-being programmes to remain in good shape (exercise routines), health food and diet, keeping your weight at the correct BMI level, and so on (Figure 7.5). It might be argued that without those aspects you would not be able to access the state's funds for social care.

Personalisation is therefore not an easy option, and could be used to reduce funding steadily over time as more and more clients or service users adopt an individual budget, whether by direct payment or using a professionally managed fund. Directing support personally (self-directed support) has the advantage of control, but it also has the disadvantage that you live with your own choices. Not everyone will want that option. Indeed, research demonstrates that while many people value highly the opportunities it creates for autonomy and freedom, there are many others for whom direct payments especially are too much trouble (for example, Clark *et al.* (2004) found take up among older people to be low and this has been confirmed subsequently). Values-based practice suggests that the users' values should be considered carefully in determining the evidence, but should also be included

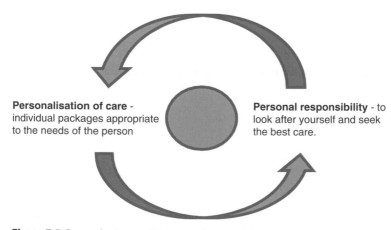

Personalisation of care - individual packages appropriate to the needs of the person

Personal responsibility - to look after yourself and seek the best care.

Figure 7.5 Personalisation requires personal responsibility.

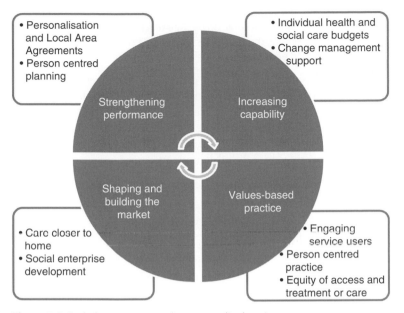

Figure 7.6 A whole-system approach to personalised services.

when it comes to deciding on the way care is to be funded. Shared decision-making is acceptable as long as it is *genuinely* shared and aggregates users' values in such a way that they are given the same status as other factors in the decision; and that decision aids are not used in effect to deny patients and service-user values by marginalising them technically in the way the aid is designed.

Figure 7.6 shows the four key building blocks of values-based individual budget arrangements (Department of Health, 2009). This demonstrates the power of individual budgets and direct payments to catalyse alternative market solutions which go beyond social care. Many private providers are considering ways to offer plural opportunities to service users with directly paid individual budgets, such that they can make available within one provider a whole range of differing packages of support relevant to the service users.

Choice is a concomitant of a strong and vibrant civic society that represents voices across all communities. By engaging *citizens* actively in a range of institutions, with locally negotiated targets of service provision, we will blur the boundaries between sectors in order to build understanding and effectiveness. The key word is citizens. We have spoken throughout the book about patients and service users, but if we want a transformative approach we need to think in terms of citizens rather than passive patients or docile service users (or, for that matter, consumers) to whom things are done. *Citizens* sums up the transformation needed: it is one of citizen choice rooted in engaged values.

As Charles Leadbeater said some years ago:

Many people's experience of being a 'consumer' is that they are put on hold, kept at arm's length, not told the whole story, tricked by the fine print, redirected to a website, treated like a number. We feel detached from large organisations – both public and private – that serve us in increasingly impersonal ways. While choice among commodity goods and services has expanded, the scope for personalised, human service, tailored to our needs, seems to have declined. (Zuboff and Maxmin, 2003 referenced in Leadbeater, 2004)

> The chasm between people and institutions is central to the future of the public sector. People may feel closely connected to and well serviced by their teacher, doctor or postman. But they often feel distant from the school, the health system or the Post Office, which they see as bureaucratic and impersonal. (Leadbeater, 2004)

A truly personalised, advanced system of social care provides support to help individual users live their lives – the support moulds around the needs and expectations of the individual. Organisational boundaries that have separated NHS care from social care, from third sector and private sector – boundaries that have never made sense to those using services – will become increasingly eroded in the future, as the complex system of care and support is attuned to the individual's needs and expectations. We need to:

- have alignment and coordination of partnerships to ensure a strategic and coordinated approach;
- use the JSNA process to include a focus on mental well-being;
- have priorities for investment and/or development;
- have investment and resource requirements in the short and medium term; and
- develop service specifications to include mental well-being and integration into existing agendas;

What is not acceptable, however, is to have a statement in a contract with the patient as follows:

> We listen to what you've got to say about your treatment, care and support. We want you to have a bigger say in how we decide whether care services are meeting essential standards.

Essential standards? We can assume that the person(s) writing this thought they were doing the right and proper thing. But on the basis that they do what they say and truly seek to understand the service user's views, setting the benchmark as 'essential standards' is very narrow, and could be made much narrower by a stroke of the pen. A genuine commitment to openness and values-based practice would say that they will listen and reflect on the service users views on 'all the care provided' and take into account the users concerns.

Dementia Care: an example

Let us consider an example (Sabat, 2011). Dementia is one of the most significant concerns faced by the population. There are estimated to be over 750,000 people in the UK with dementia and numbers are expected to double in the next 30 years. 'Dementia' is used to describe a syndrome which may be caused by a number of illnesses in which there is progressive decline in multiple areas of function. Although dementia is primarily a condition associated with older people, there are also a significant number of people (currently around 15,000) who develop dementia earlier in life. Of all people with dementia among Black and minority ethnic (BME) groups, 6.1% have early-onset dementia, compared with only 2.2% for the UK population as a whole, reflecting the younger age profile of BME communities. Direct costs of dementia to the NHS and Social Care are in the region of £8.2 billion annually. The national strategy was followed in November 2009 by the publication of a report addressing the over-prescription of antipsychotic medication for people with dementia. Implementation of the 11 recommendations contained within that report is an integral part of improving the care and experience of people with dementia and their carers.

'Living Well With Dementia' (the national dementia strategy) 2009 is being implemented over a five-year period to 2014. It sets out 17 objectives for transforming dementia services, with the aim of accelerating the pace of improvement in dementia care, through local delivery of quality outcomes and local accountability for achieving them. This new outcomes-focused approach will ensure greater transparency and provision of information to individuals, enabling people to have a good understanding of their local services, how these compare to other services, and the level of quality that they can expect. Within the strategy are a number of important components: work being done by the Department of Health on quality and outcomes; work by the national Alzheimer's Disease Society; and work by NICE. NICE set itself the challenge of developing guidance that is both evidence-based and draws on the views and wishes of 'ordinary' people. It has a well-designed process of consultation, but recognises that not all its efforts to engage communities will be successful, although it has used patient or service-user groups to comment on and to discuss its findings.

The stage of the pathway that is of interest is on 'principles of care' (NICE/SCIE, 2006). The list of points is important and will ensure, if followed, that the person is dealt with more or less appropriately. They include: always treating people with dementia and their carers with respect; ensuring that people with dementia are not excluded from services because of their diagnosis, age, or any learning disability; provision of information in an appropriate language; ensuring that people suspected of having dementia because of cognitive and functional deterioration, but who do not have sufficient memory impairment for diagnosis, are not denied access to support services; identifying specific needs including those arising from diversity (such as sex, ethnicity, age, religion and personal care), or co-morbidities, physical and learning disabilities, sensory impairment, communication difficulties, problems with nutrition and poor oral health. Additionally, NICE stress the importance of consent and capacity, focusing on the use of the Mental Capacity Act if loss of capacity is suspected and recognising the position of advance statements, advance decisions to refuse treatment, Lasting Powers of Attorney and a Preferred Place of Care Plan. The impact of dementia on personal (including sexual) relationships and safeguarding are noted, as is the possibility of individual budget and direct payments.

Diversity and equality, language and interpretation, needs and preferences, ethics and consent, and advocacy are all considered in some depth. Even then, there are values that might be relevant that have not been taken into account. For instance, what operational policy does the hospital have for ensuring that a person is able at all times to obtain necessary food and drink? What opportunities are offered for living as independently as possible, perhaps in a separate room in the nursing home? What opportunities are provided to meet the ethnic preferences of residents? What audit arrangements to involve carers have been made?

While the NICE guidelines suggest a wide range of questions, the way in which hospitals and nursing homes meet these requirements varies enormously. Who will ensure that the person is treated correctly once in care? How will a nursing home know what to provide for someone from a minority ethnic background or minority faith? Will there be consistency in providing care? It is apparent from the Good Practice Compendium that each area and place of good practice has developed options for and is achieving services to meet part but not all needs. An holistic response is needed that recognises the values of (a) the population of all those with dementia and their carers, and (b) the needs of individual patients.

Understanding the religious values of the person may challenge commissioners to seek alternative providers that can intelligently and sensitively offer tailor-made services to clients from a minority religion, community or culture. This is essential now, but will become more and more necessary over time as minority communities age and older people suffer from dementia. It is not sufficient to say that there are so few people from a particular religion that their needs cannot be met. However, information on dementia in minority communities is very limited. They may want different facilities, such as to be able to wash in running water, and they may want these in nursing and care homes that offer high-quality care to everyone. The number of people with dementia in minority ethnic groups is estimated to be around 15,000 in England – approximately 3% of the estimated overall number of people with dementia, and the number of people from ethnic minorities with dementia, and their proportion of the population as a whole, is set to rise quickly (Equality Impact Assessment, for Living well with dementia, National Dementia Strategy). There is some evidence that some minority ethnic groups may have higher levels of early onset dementia, in their thirties and forties, and will require a heightened response (Blackburn Local Council, personal communication). Dementia is progressive and it is often unclear when a person has reached a threshold that may lead to danger or neglect. The use of psychotic medication is one element in treatment (see above).

However, the principles do not extend to problems posed by cognitive impairment as a result of the illness and the ever present danger of wandering, seeking old and familiar surroundings, or acting on memories from years gone by. Some patients become aggressive at times; the service must have mechanisms for managing patients effectively in ways that recognise their inherent worth and humanity. The stigma and abbreviated autonomy that is implied in managing people with dementia requires a new holistic method of managing their care that relates the care to the patients'/service users' values. This is nowhere more evident than in long-term care, where: '[L]eaving aside whether these terms have any particular diagnostic validity in particular cases, the fact that an individual's life can be readily reconstituted and reduced through the foreshortening effect of such labels raises obvious questions about the effects of biography on autonomy' (Agich, 1993).

Cultural and social differences may be an obstacle for some ethnic minority communities accessing health and social care. For example, there is no word for dementia in five South Asian languages; even if there is good translation, it does not ensure that what is translated is understood. More importantly, there are value-based differences that may become serious barriers to the provision of adequate care. In Gujurati communities, an older man with capacity will defer to his son, but professional staff may insist that they talk only to the older person (Shah, personal communication). People of South Asian heritage may recognise symptoms associated with dementia, but not think of these as part of an illness even when they are severe (Lawrence *et al.*, 2008).

Other values that prevent BME patients and family members from engaging with formal services include the belief that 'nothing can be done, a lack of awareness of available services, a lack of awareness of access procedures for available services, the belief that available services are inadequate, inaccessible and culturally insensitive, previous poor experience of services and stigma attached to mental disorder' (Equality Impact Assessment, for Living well with dementia, National Dementia Strategy). Many of the present generation of minority ethnic elders came to the UK as adults, and many have not acquired fluency or literacy in English. Any diagnostic or social tests requiring numeracy, literacy or cultural understanding may be difficult if not impossible for them.

Values and outcomes

As we saw in Chapter 4, by recognising a person's values it is possible to construct the outcome(s) that will satisfy his or her goals. Some of those values may be narrowly medical, but a wider set will describe the outcome of care from a holistic viewpoint (Figure 7.7).

Values-based practice suggests that the critical issue is the outcome goal to be achieved, which in turn is informed by the values of the patient or service user. By working

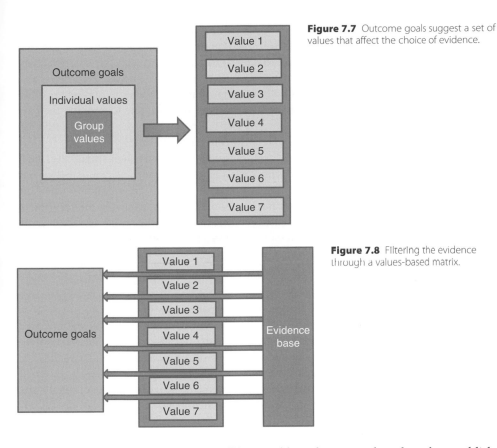

Figure 7.7 Outcome goals suggest a set of values that affect the choice of evidence.

Figure 7.8 Filtering the evidence through a values-based matrix.

backwards from the outcome goal it will be possible to determine the values that established that goal, and thus create a filter for the evidence (Figure 7.8). The evidence available should be filtered through the values matrix as established to inform best practice for one or more patients.

Filtering in this way is not easy. It demands knowledge of a set of values (and these will differ depending on the issue at hand), and the ability to take the evidence and filter it as suggested. That in turn requires a careful analysis of the data in such a way that the patient's outcome goal is accessible from the treatment or service provided. One way of doing this is through the process of deciding personal health and social care budgets.

Personal health and social care budgets

Personal health and/or social care budgets will begin to change the way that health systems and social care provision are made. By determining the patients' or the service users'/clients' values, beliefs and preferences, it will be possible to describe a service that draws on those values for its structure and purpose. Some service users may be given a budget held by the professional staff of social care; others may have a direct payment. Similarly this will develop in health care, especially for people with long-term or progressive disorders that can be managed in the community. By understanding the values of the patients and service users we can construct outcome goals and work back to a prescription of the service that meets those goals in ways that are acceptable to the service user and come within a cost demanded by the service.

Complex nursing and social care at home or in institutions is cost-determined rather than values-determined. Wanting to remain in your own home is a values-based matter, but that may or may not be possible. Being required to move into a large (and relatively cost-effective) care home may be one option over which you have no control and little say; but conversely, being required to stay in your own home without proper care and attention may be the other lower-cost option. It may be convenient or inconvenient for the state to provide the care there: it may be more expensive or less expensive depending on a range of factors, although largely on whether you have an informal carer who will cost very little.

How far can your values outweigh these considerations? To what extent should the carers who come into *your* home have to put up with your way of life (your mess, your smells, your smoke, your swearing!)? To what extent should I have to abandon my autonomy when the state says that I need my care provision in a nursing home? If we are to ensure the very best at a time of austerity we need a values-based discussion in depth with every service user, to understand what is most important or pressing, and what might be lost by mutual agreement in determining the care package.

Conclusion

Integrative care offers the option of bringing together elements of care from a variety of sources. However, as we have said previously, that should be following a full values-based exercise that ensures there is good communication and an understanding both ways of values (my values, and professional values), and a recognition of the evidence as far as we have it, filtered or reflected through our values. When we describe care pathways we must recognise that they are not linear: patients and service users traverse these pathways in complex ways. By person-centring the care pathway we will recognise the inherent variability of need. Only by addressing that need through the lens of patient or service user values will it be possible to achieve a genuinely personalised care.

Priority setting and resource allocation: values, ethics, evidence

Introduction

After a discussion of behaviour changes associated with the establishment of Clinical Commissioning Groups (although not directly the domain of this book), possibly the most important aspect of any systemic change is the way that priority-setting and resource allocation is undertaken. An ethically based resource allocation procedure for decision-making at times of financial pressure is an essential toolkit for any commissioning management. Although there is a lot to be done to set up CCGs and the other aspects of the government's proposed changes to the health and social care system, the need for a robust and ethical resource allocation system is unarguable. Unfortunately, with so many changes to the overall system, and with the harsh austerity measures beginning to bite, it is likely that commissioners will make quick and sometimes erroneous judgements about resources that may be, at best, less than optimal, and at worst leave some patients with poorer care than previously.

Under the previous regime the 11 World Class Commissioning (WCC) competencies contained two competencies that were especially relevant to priority setting and resource allocation.

- Competency 6: prioritise investment according to local needs, service requirements and the values of the NHS. 'By having a clear understanding of the needs of different sections of the local population, PCTs, with their partners, will set strategic priorities and make investment decisions, focused on the achievement of key clinical and health and community outcomes. This will include investment plans that address the areas of greatest health inequality'.

- Competency 11: make sound financial investments to ensure sustainable developments and value for money. PCTs will ensure that their commissioning decisions are sustainable and provide a sound investment to secure improved health outcomes for both now and the future. Excellent financial skills and clinical resource management will enable PCTs to manage the financial risks involved in commissioning, and to take a proactive rather than reactive approach to financial management. The financial strategy will ensure that the commissioning strategy is affordable and set within the organisation's overall risk and assurance framework. (Department of Health, 2007.)

These competencies can be mapped directly onto clinical commissioning groups. Competency 6 required PCTs (now PCT clusters) and CCGs, supported by clinical senates and the national Commissioning Board, and by extension Health and Well-being Boards and social care providers, to develop processes to measure needs (and assets), to establish priorities for investment in health care, and to tackle health inequalities; and competency 11 requires CCGs and other to have the financial management processes in place to ensure adequate and acceptable standards and risk profiles. While unexceptional, these two competencies, however devised or written, explain the importance of a good, ethically driven resource allocation system that is, and can be shown to be, robust, well-designed, dynamic and influential.

Setting priorities in health and social care is possibly one of the most difficult things that commissioners can do. Although the management and leadership of public organisations and the development of commissioning processes is challenging enough, deciding on the proper use of resources is fraught with problems. The critical and most contentious decisions that any commissioning body can take are those that offer or deny particular treatments for certain conditions within a context that requires, ethically, socially, and politically, the most cost- and clinically effective use of those resources. There is never enough money; and that fact alone, in practice, exposes to scrutiny, argument and challenge the values of all those involved in the process.

Similarly, good resource allocation demands a transparent, albeit complex process. Allocating resources fairly requires a priority-setting procedure that is multi-factorial, multi-ethnic and multi-faith and crucially recognises and identifies differences of values. Priority-setting and resource allocation throws up a constant stream of 'wicked problems' that demand thoughtful, values-based answers that are defensible because they are determined by explicit values made transparent, and based on due process, in which differing trade-offs have been identified and explored (see, for example, Chang, 1997). In short, priority setting is a values-based activity (see, for example, Seedhouse, 2005).

Resource allocation

A strong resource allocation process will:

- use robust evidence and public health intelligence to plan and commission services;
- ensure a 'full-blooded' values process and analysis;
- aim to achieve full engagement of the public, patients, service users and other stakeholders;
- use care or clinical pathways as the basis for whole-systems design;
- enter into committed partnerships with providers, primary care teams, patients and service user groups and other stakeholders;
- take a whole-systems perspective recognising the inter-related aspects of primary health and social care with secondary (and tertiary) acute medicine and surgery and other services (as we saw in relation to whole systems);
- work with providers on innovative ways to use resources to maximum benefit and to recognise that commissioning is a 'two-way street' – i.e. between commissioners and providers; and
- balance the investment across the spectrum of health and social care from complex (expensive) acute medical and surgical cases (e.g. whole bowel transplants), to complex (expensive) cases in the community (e.g. continuing care for very disabled people at home).

The purpose of this chapter is thus threefold: to offer an ethical framework that will enable difficult priority-setting decisions to be made at a time of financial constraint; to catalyse further discussion about the most appropriate process to be adopted by PCTs, CCGs, Health and Well-being Boards and others; and to ensure that new systems build on good practice and values as a firm foundation for establishing priority-setting and resource-allocation procedures.

Values-based practice is an essential aspect of resource allocation. The values of the individual, group, community and population will have an impact to a greater or lesser extent. Understanding those values and finding ways to negotiate values will be crucial to informed debate and the results that are obtained. This demands due process, even if that were not a legal requirement, and mechanisms for involving the public, patients and service users meaningfully in the process of decision-making; it offers pointers to an acceptable, although complex, mechanism that merges and amalgamates a variety of processes.

An essential aspect of an effective priority-setting process is that it must have as much certainty as possible about what it wants to achieve – the aims and objectives commissioners set for a resource-allocation procedure. Some commissioners may want to seek to achieve a 'root and branch' review of what is funded – i.e. what it 'offers' to the public and patients, and by extension what it demands of providers. Undertaking such a review may require a zero-based budgeting exercise to understand the basis of all health care expenditure. Although this may seem daunting, it is probable that the financial position will require something like this to be done in many places if fairness and equity are to be preserved. Second, some commissioners may want to retain a process for making investment and disinvestment at the margins, thus more-or-less taking as read that most services should be, and indeed can only be amended a little from year to year. This is sometimes described as limited list prioritisation, best undertaken using PBMA. Third, others may not want, initially at least, to become embroiled in discussions on significant changes and will prefer to prepare a set of values and guidelines to give context to any difficult resource allocation decision but not to have a specific or detailed procedure for priority-setting.

These three possibilities lie on a spectrum of opportunities that set the ground rules for the activity; they are not the only options. The process could develop a 'core offer' that delivers 'best value' for the community and enables marginal changes to be handled in a firm context of agreed overall provision. No process can or will provide the 'correct' answer. Priority setting is complex and defies simple solutions. However, it is essential to develop a process that is 'good enough' and 'fit for purpose', that addresses the aims and objectives of commissioners and the public, reflects the reality of the financial constraints, and is acceptable – in other words, has face validity as perceived by the ordinary patient or service user. In developing this process, it may be necessary for a robust argument within the NHS and local authorities about the constraints and to challenge the accepted wisdom on what is a good health outcome.

As the system becomes more complex – with CCGs, Health and Well-being Boards, PCT clusters, clinical senates and the National Commissioning Board – many commissioners may wish to keep the process simple and practical, partly as a result of resource constraints, but more particularly because initially at least there will be a lot of guidance from the centre at a time of severe cash shortages. Making the process more complicated is unlikely to appeal to busy GPs. Having said that, the time to invest in values-based commissioning is at the beginning, to set in place a process that establishes how a CCG wishes to continue, and to obtain patient and public values, regularly and comprehensively, using all means available.

This may lead to further radical proposals to change health (and social care) targets. Do national tariffs make sense in all aspects of healthcare when local conditions need to be reflected more fully? Should there be greater freedom to determine local priorities even if these conflict with national targets? Indeed, it has been argued that targets may affect resource-allocation decisions if their achievement results in some patients that are not the subject of targets being treated unfairly (UK Clinical Ethics Network). Other questions may arise as a better resource-allocation system is developed.

Ethical robustness

A priority-setting or resource-allocation system will not be ethical or acceptable if it is not accompanied by a sustained effort to use all available resources in the most effective, efficient and economical way. One of the problems of limited list marginal investment processes is that they do not consider the whole investment 'in the round'. Denying one set of patients the new drug(s) that may improve the quality or save their life, but allowing waste in the system somewhere else, is neither ethically sound nor practical politics. There are many ways in which costs can be saved without tough priority decisions. These include, for example, utilisation management, referral threshold management, efficient use of plant, and use of the most cost- and clinically efficient and effective treatment.

What matters is to recognise that investment and disinvestment go hand in hand. Providers should be asked to engage in a process for determining the best use of resources for existing services at the same time as identifying new ways of working that use the available resources to maximum patient benefit. Commissioners must at once balance investment in prevention and intervention, address health inequalities as well as immediate health need, tackle efficiency and waste, seek to add 'life to years and years to life', improve overall health outcomes, and offer an increasingly personalised service that meets individual need in the most effective way. This has to be done at a time of very serious reduction in real terms of funding of the NHS and local government, increasing treatment costs such as new medicines, significant demographic shifts such as the increasing numbers of elderly and very elderly people in society, and the impact of national priorities and central guidance, such as NICE guidelines.

The policy should describe first (philosophical) principles – for example, the four fundamental principles (Beauchamp and Childress, 2001), and process principles such as 'Accountability for Reasonableness' (Daniels, 2000; Daniels and Sabin, 1997), and ensure that this offers a good platform on which to build a comprehensive resource allocation programme. These principles are then used to frame a process of programme budgeting using cost–utility or cost-effectiveness criteria. The work by Peter Brambleby, Muir Gray and others has demonstrated the value of PBMA as an important tool of priority setting and resource allocation. The best paper to recommend, which captures all the detail that would otherwise be in this chapter, is the 'Third Annual Population Review: Commissioning for Health Improvement: Using programme budgeting and marginal analysis to deliver quality, innovation productivity and prevention' (Brambleby et al., 2010). This report describes fully the various techniques that can be used to give full effect to PBMA-driven resource allocation and covers much that is hinted at here. With one exception: it does not place an emphasis on values and values-based commissioning.

Whatever system is used must provide the rigour to make some tough decisions about the overall balance of health and social care. Many PCTs historically have used limited list marginal investment systems without recognising the holistic nature of health and social care. One problem with an encompassing system of this type is that it can be manipulated to give almost any answer. It provides a good basis for discussion of the options and demands some rigour, for example in requiring evidence of the effectiveness of interventions, but does not put sufficient weight on cost–benefit analysis, or programme budget comparators. Listing investment decisions in resource allocation order without reference to cost can lead to perverse decisions (unless the cost–benefit or cost–utility [cost per QALY and QALYs gained per unit of investment]) of all options are calculated rigorously.

Critical concerns

A tough resource-allocation process must recognise certain practical constraints and not succumb to the myth that commissioners have more than a marginal effect on the resource allocation outcome in any one year, unless they are prepared to look at the total spend in a much more radical way. For example, it is very difficult to move more than 1–2% of the budget in any one year. Even that is a challenge unless commissioners are enormously courageous; 3% of a Foundation Trust budget of, say, £300 million is £9 million. That is roughly the maximum saving from a cost improvement programme. Commissioners are generally not good at innovating on their own but need providers to work with them. Commissioning (and thus resource allocation) is a two-way street! Most of the health commissioners' budget is spent by GPs. GPs make thousands of decisions every week that determine where the patients and thus the money goes. Unless they are engaged fully with this process, understand the reasons for decisions and accept the rationale for them, no resource-allocation process will work and much of the debate will be a waste of time.

Aristotle helpfully set out the problem 2500 years ago. In the Nichomachean Ethics he said, more or less, 'treat equals equally and un-equals unequally in proportion to their relevant difference' (Aristotle, 2000). This Aristotelian formulation helpfully describes the problem, but only goes a short way to offering a solution. Clarity about equity is essential, although even then what we mean by equity is itself a potential problem. The literature contains many differing definitions. Do we mean equality of concern and respect for each individual, or equity of resource input, or equity of outcome, or equality of ability to benefit? How do we achieve equity in 'adding life to years and years to life' (i.e. in tackling health inequalities) while at the same time meeting immediate, perhaps very expensive, life-saving procedures? The NHS has for many years been an illness service rather than a health service. As we place greater emphasis on tackling prevention, well-being, lifestyle and inequalities, how do we balance the short-term demands with the longer-term strategy to improve population health? Similarly, how do we achieve equity between competing demands?

The framework for priority-setting and resource allocation should incorporate important ethical principles, considerations of due process, with a set of practical procedures based on experience of 'what works'. The ethical issues can be described in four domains (see the box below), to which should be added reasonable, justifiable and acceptable procedures, and engagement and involvement of the general public, patients, service users and other recipients of health (and social) care, and stakeholders from the communities served: once there is agreement to these ethical domains and process elements it is then possible to identify sound practical procedures that are based on lessons learned from the many attempts over the previous 20 years to develop effective resource-allocation procedures, that may be suited to the PCT or that have special relevance or resonance locally.

Table 8.1 Elements of a robust process for priority-setting.

Part	Description	Notes
1 Decision on ethical objectives	The ethical constructs that frame the decision process. This includes decisions on national targets; meeting local objectives, policy on addressing health inequalities, and wider benefits to society	Generic requirement of any procedure
2 Decision on cost–benefit	PBMA processes focus on programme categories and look at comparative spend with similar CCGs or PCTs. Includes the availability and strength of evidence, the magnitude of realisable benefit, the number who will benefit (the wider benefit not necessarily the number treated), and the total cost of the investment	Individual programme areas. Can be done separately in a phased programme
3 Decision on alternatives	Individual condition–treatment options for specific conditions where there is good evidence that an alternative treatment or intervention may be more cost or clinically effective. Could be based on care pathways, as the way of identifying the most appropriate and cost effective pathway, and bringing providers (NHS, local authority, private and not-for-profit) into consideration	Individual cost-effectiveness process or a separate marginal investment process
4 Decision on social determinant	Comparison across programme groups to ensure equity taking into account the CCG, PCT cluster, or Health and Well-being Board decision on social determinants of health; could be used as part of a radical review and zero-based budgeting scheme	Radical review

In order to achieve a comprehensive approach to priority-setting, we need a process that offers something to each of these elements, and incorporates the values of patients and service users into the bargain (see Table 8.1).

Fundamental rights and freedoms: ethical concerns for a flourishing, safe human society

Any health care resource-allocation process should espouse fundamental ethical principles of a good society. We might argue about the scope and extent of these principles, but they will include those set out in the Universal Declaration of Human Rights, the European Convention on Human Rights and similar internationally agreed conventions and instruments. These are well summed up in the phrase 'life, liberty and the pursuit of happiness',[1] or perhaps should also include well-being. The right to life, something we espouse as a fundamental building block of a modern society, is in fact problematic in health care. Commissioners should consider what this means for any resource-allocation criteria. Is 'life' rather than 'quality of life' the main goal, regardless of cost or suffering? This becomes

---

[1] One of the most famous quotations from the US Declaration of Independence. These are inalienable rights and thus set an ethical benchmark. Probably John Locke as described by Curry (2011): 'no one ought to harm another in his life, health, liberty, or possessions.' An alternative source is Blackstone's Commentaries on the Laws of England (1753, Introduction, section 2, of the Nature of Laws in General).

especially relevant in dealing with end-of-life concerns. To what extent do we 'strive officiously to keep alive'? More importantly, can commissioners, in conversation with the public and stakeholders, put some boundaries on those interventions that will or will not be funded towards or at the end of life? These are tricky questions as they can generate a great deal of emotion and fear, but they have to be addressed if commissioners are to control expenditure in a way that is acceptable to the public.

Taking a human rights perspective on health care resource allocation forces us to address the implications of other clauses of the Universal Declaration on Human Rights (UDHR) or the European Convention on Human Rights (ECHR).[2] For example, the right to private and family life should be borne in mind at all times when considering the best way to provide care for physically disabled people.

General ethical principles (that are particularly suited to health care)

Each of the four principles below is important in the provision of health care, but these principles are also valuable in providing a robust context for resource allocation. A great deal of debate during the past 10 years has centred on 'principalism' versus other ethical tenets, such as human rights or rule-based systems. While a simple reliance on a set of a-priori principles may not be sufficient for a fully functioning ethical framework, they do nonetheless provide a valuable context and point to important questions that must be considered (Beauchamp and Childress, 2011). The points made below in italics are questions that require answers; a commissioner must be able to give a good account for each of these questions.

- Respect for autonomy: respecting the decision-making capacities of autonomous persons; enabling individuals to make reasoned and informed choices. *How is choice reflected adequately in allocative systems? How are individuals' needs considered in the context of wider population need? What level of choice will commissioners allow? To what extent will individuals be able to shape their own care or care packages?*

- Beneficence: considers the balancing of benefits of treatment against the risks and costs; the healthcare (or social care) professional should act always in a way that benefits the patient. *The balance required here is relevant to equity and assertive mechanisms to address health inequalities. What imperative do commissioners wish to place on addressing health inequalities? What system for addressing health inequalities is needed? Is it to level up or level down?*

---

[2] Article 3. Everyone has the right to life, liberty and security of person.
Article 4. No one shall be held in slavery or servitude; slavery and the slave trade shall be prohibited in all their forms.
Article 5. No one shall be subjected to torture or to cruel, inhuman or degrading treatment or punishment.
Article 6. Everyone has the right to recognition everywhere as a person before the law.
Article 7. All are equal before the law and are entitled without any discrimination to equal protection of the law. All are entitled to equal protection against any discrimination in violation of this Declaration and against any incitement to such discrimination.

- Non-malfeasance: avoiding the causation of harm; the health or social care professional should not harm the patient. All treatment involves some harm (and collective medical or social care cause some harms to those denied certain treatment or support), even if minimal, but the harm should not be disproportionate to the benefits of treatment. *What harm will be done if resources are not allocated fairly or proportionate to need? Can the commissioners (with providers) identify the harms that may be caused if funding for existing services is reduced or withdrawn?*

- Justice: distributing benefits, risks and costs fairly; the notion that patients or service users in similar positions should be treated in a similar manner (see the Aristotelian formula above). *Justice as fairness is an essentially contested concept! What system of just allocation will the commissioners wish to adopt? In particular, will commissioners wish to ensure, as far as possible, equal ability to benefit? Or will commissioners want a different principle to apply, such as equity of inputs or outcomes?*

Ethically relevant economic principles

Any resource-allocation system will use some form of economic analysis, in the main rooted in utilitarianism (Drummond *et al.*, 1987; Hoffmann *et al.*, 2002). By this we mean systems that have the objective of maximising population health or healthy gain. Such utilitarian mechanisms ensure a focus on cost or cost–benefit but may not ensure that other important imperatives of a resource-allocation system are given sufficient weight. A good resource-allocation system will ensure a balance between utilitarian (economic) analyses and rule- or rights-based imperatives.

Utilitarian approaches to health resource allocation have the advantage of focusing on maximising health gain, but there is the danger that they may support resources being allocated to less-expensive treatments or services that provide the greatest overall benefit (Pettiti, 2011). Utilitarianism does not take into account the population 'need' for the healthcare intervention and relies rather on an equation of cost and the effectiveness of treatment. While cost–benefit or cost-effectiveness *must* be one of the criteria of good resource allocation, it is important to recognise the built in 'discrimination error' that biases decisions in favour of prevention over intervention, or interventions that achieve identified health gain over those that address health inequalities. As important is the need to understand the population values if a utilitarian perspective is to be acceptable, but then we have to account for differing ethical positions, such as those of minority groups.

Three main forms of economic evaluation are used: cost-effectiveness analysis, cost–benefit analysis, and cost–utility analysis (Mitton and Donaldson, 2004).

- Cost-effectiveness analysis (CEA) is used to address questions of technical efficiency where a choice needs to be made between two options with the same already determined objective.

- Cost–benefit analysis (CBA) is concerned predominantly to assess which goals or objectives may be worth achieving – more directly, how much resource to allocate to a particular type of healthcare.

- Cost–utility analysis (CUA) can be used to tackle technical or evaluative efficiency.

Depending on the definitions used and the resource allocation process,[3] there will be overlaps between these options. The best known cost–utility application is the use of Quality Adjusted Life Years (QALYs) as a means of comparing the net benefit from healthcare interventions. Healthcare effectiveness is measured by both increased life expectancy and the increased quality of life (adding 'years to life and life to years'), achieved by the intervention. At first blush this seems to be both attractive and relatively objective. Unfortunately, there have been many criticisms of QALYs, not least that the scales used in QALY calculations are based on small-scale research samples which contain significant value judgements. The genesis of QALY calculations should be made explicit as they may not be relevant to the population that a commissioner is assessing (Harris, 1987). Because QALYs are so value-laden, the utility of the cost–utility equation demands careful consideration. Engaging patients and service users to reflect specifically on the utility aspect of these calculations may generate a different set of weights to those used in the literature. In doing so, commissioners may find challenges to the accepted outcomes from published accounts, and may wish to make changes appropriately.

There are, however, a number of differing definitions of utility in the literature. Two are particularly interesting: as an individual's feeling of wellness, or as an expression of the value an individual assigns to her state of health (Nord, 1999). Nord argues that these are conceptually different, but are they? Nord describes the first as the 'quantity of wellness interpretation', what he refers to as an emotional category; and the second as a 'value interpretation', a cognitive category. Despite a sophisticated argument about using expected utility theory to account for the former, and time trade-off (and the more complicated standard gamble) for the latter, at root the two are both evaluative concepts. They are not 'facts', but values, dressed in different clothes but values nonetheless. What this suggests is that cost–value and cost–utility theory rests on a powerfully *evaluative* programme, which in turn both underpins our contention about the importance of 'values', and demonstrates that much 'objective' assessment of the evidence will simply not wash.

Many healthcare interventions are not the subject of a QALY assessment and direct comparisons between the cost–benefit of different treatments is not possible. QALYs by definition are based on population-level information and do not take into account individual

---

[3] Technical efficiency: for a given input, maximise

- output
- health
- survival
- quality of life
- benefit or utility

    Productive efficiency: minimise cost

- at maximum output
- per unit of survival
- per QALY

    Allocative efficiency

- maximise value at given cost
- ensure right mix of outputs for competing outcomes

response to illness; they are inherently ageist, although this assertion is contentious, and they may discriminate against people with disabilities and congenital abnormalities (see Hope *et al.*, 2003; Lockwood, 1988). An alternative approach is to use Disability Adjusted Life Years (DALYs) – a measure of the burden of disease on a defined population and the effectiveness of interventions (Last, 2006).

DALYs are advocated as an alternative to QALYs and claimed to be a valid indicator of population health (World Bank, 1993). They are based on adjustment of life expectancy to allow for long-term disability as estimated from official statistics. However, their use as currently expressed and calculated may be limited because the necessary data are not available or do not exist. Moreover, the concept postulates a continuum from disease to disability to death that is not universally accepted, particularly by the community of persons with disabilities. DALYs are calculated using a 'disability weight' (a proportion less than 1 multiplied by chronological age to reflect the burden of the disability) which can thus produce estimates that accord greater value to fit than to disabled persons, and to the middle years of life rather than to youth or old age (Arnesen and Nord, 1999).

Economic considerations are at the heart of PBMA, a technique for comparing the costs and outcomes of broad programmes of health care. PBMA has the advantage of simplicity, directness, and offers a way of fairly objectively addressing horizontal equity concerns (see below). However, it does not address matters of rights or recognition or equity unless these are explicitly imported into the process. Values-based practice offers the chance to engage service users more fully in discussion of the fundamental aspects of PBMA, on the values that should be incorporated, and thus of the results that emerge.

Evidence and values come together in determining QALY figures. There is no such thing as an objective assessment of utility. It is a subjective assessment of how an individual feels about the care provided and the outcomes it achieves from the point of view of the patient or service user. The only claim to neutrality is where there are sufficient subjects that the individual preferences are ironed out statistically, but they are values not evidence, despite claims that we can turn values into evidence. QALY calculations come as close as anything to an amalgam of evidence (which has other values associated with it) and values as assessed utility.

Equity

Aristotle's 'formal principle of equality' provides a good description of the resource-allocation problem. Although it does not solve the problem, it demands that criteria are set out explicitly for what we mean by equal and unequal. Aristotle's own criteria were based on merit; in the twenty-first century 'merit' in health care should usually mean clinical need. (The utilitarian or QALY based approach could be said to treat un-equals equally, in that it does not take account of differences in need for health care but focuses entirely on the benefit gained from an intervention.) Allocative and 'political' principles such as equity, recognition and justice should ensure that treatment is made available according to need.

Some individuals or groups of patients will have poorer health than others, or more serious diseases, and will have a greater need of health care. If degree of need is a main criterion, a just distribution of health care resources may require that these individuals or groups have more resources, even if the benefit gained by treatment is small compared to that achieved by a different treatment in patients that are less sick. In other words, any resource-allocation scheme should take account affirmatively of social determinants of health and pre-existing circumstances outside the patient's control (see, for example, the UK Clinical Ethics Network, Ethox Centre, University of Oxford).

Many philosophers have offered theories of justice that may be relevant to health care. One that has been particularly influential is John Rawls' 'Theory of Justice' (1971). For Rawls, a just allocation of resources will be one that, all other things being equal, benefits the worst off in society. This is a 'strong' value. Thus, in the context of health care we should allocate resources to ensure that those in poorest health, or greatest need, are as well off in terms of health as they can be. Others see justice as necessarily reflecting previous injustices, prior discrimination and recognition of equal human worth (Sen, 2009; Franklin, 1998). This is echoed by Fraser and Honneth (2003), who contend that social justice and self-realisation are essential goals of a system of resource allocation – recognition of difference is itself a necessary feature of allocative processes (Harris, 1995).

Reducing health inequalities is now accepted as a key aim of the NHS. This comes in broadly three forms: first, those inequalities that arise from specific decisions of the NHS to invest in one treatment rather than another or to allow different levels of treatment in different geographical areas; second, from the problems of horizontal equity – ensuring that unlike disease groups have more or less similar access to a range of necessary and appropriate treatments; and third (and more importantly in this case), from social determinants of health. Addressing the needs of disadvantaged groups or minority communities with specific and unrecognised need is paramount.

Any differences between individuals or groups that are used to justify different treatment must be morally relevant differences. That might seem to suggest that factors such as ethnicity, sex, or income are not relevant, but discrimination based on these factors has been and continues to be a problem. Minority ethnic groups have had worse healthcare for many years, either because of language or education leading to reduced access, or deliberate discrimination on the basis of race, or as a result of lower investment in necessary services (such as sickle cell disease for Black Africans). Where there has been systematic discrimination (whether intentional or not) over a long period of time on grounds of ethnicity, gender, faith, age, disability or any other ground over which a person (or persons) has no control, then the resource-allocation mechanism should seek to take affirmative action to tackle the resultant health inequalities. This again is a 'strong' value, which requires the interrogation of wider community values, and a negotiation about its relevance and impact.

Due process, reasonable, justifiable and acceptable procedures

R v North West Lancashire Health Authority ex parte A, D and G (1999) 53 BMLR 148, [2000] 1 WLR 977

The Court of Appeal said that a decision regarding the provision of treatment must be taken within a proper framework. Although it is appropriate for a Health Authority *(and thus PCT or other relevant authority)* to have a policy for establishing certain priorities in funding different treatments, in establishing priorities – comparing respective needs of patients suffering from different illnesses and determining the respective strengths of their claims to treatment – it is vital for the Health Authority to:

- accurately assess the nature and seriousness of each type of illness;
- determine the effectiveness of various forms of treatment for it; and
- give proper effect to that assessment and that determination in the formulation and individual application of its policy.

Accountability for reasonableness

As the quotation above suggests, due process in priority-setting and resource allocation is essential. This has been tested many times in the Courts. There is (by and large) no right to a specific healthcare intervention or service under the NHS Acts, but there is a presumption that any decision is taken following proper and careful consideration, and that the process is transparent.

Norman Daniels and Jim Sabin (2002) at Harvard, building on Rawls, suggested a process that they called 'accountability for reasonableness'. Although rooted in North American experience it has been accepted internationally as a benchmark of good process. The four tenets are:

- *publicity* – decisions and their rationales must be publicly accessible;
- *reasonableness* – the rationales for decisions should appeal to reasons and principles that are accepted as relevant by people who are prepared to look for mutually agreeable and culturally acceptable forms of engagement;
- *appeals* – there is a mechanism for challenge and dispute resolution; and
- *enforcement* – there is either voluntary or public regulation of the process.

Although these provide a sound basis, they are not uncontentious. Transparency is to be welcomed, but to be effective the process and information about the process and its outcome must be available to all. 'Reasonableness' begs the question of whose reasonableness, which may differ depending on the community or culture in which decisions are taken. An appeals mechanism must be fair but not allow a coach and horses to be driven through well-chosen decisions after careful deliberation; and enforcement must be just that – if commissioners take tough decisions, they should see them through.

As Daniels and Sabin place a premium on reasonableness, it is acceptable for us to ask whose values go to make up what is 'reasonable'. Their formulation is an appeal to 'reasons and principles that are accepted as relevant by people who are prepared to look for mutually agreeable and culturally acceptable forms of engagement'. This suggests at least two challenges that lead to a relativism in the outcome: how is a mutual agreement achieved, and how do we achieve cultural acceptability. By and large, their formulation is akin to Rawls' 'original position', which unashamedly contains North American liberal values. It does not take into account sufficiently the differing perspectives and values in the USA, let alone Europe.

Obtaining mutual agreement requires a values-based discussion identifying those values where the 'wheel squeaks', where there is a difference of values on which the work is done. Mutual agreement between all stakeholders may be impossible, and it may be necessary to agree to differ – to have dissonance – such that there is more than one policy or resource-allocation position. It may require a suite of decisions that are appropriate for different groups in society; and this may be permissible if the differences are large enough or of importance to stakeholders. Similarly, cultural acceptability may take many forms and may lead to different expressions of policy.

However, 'accountability for reasonableness' is a process measure. The mutual agreement and cultural acceptability refers to 'forms of engagement', not to the substance of the result, but how can we have mutually agreeable and culturally acceptable forms of engagement, and not have mutually agreeable and culturally acceptable results? By accepting this form of procedural rationality, we articulate the need for a multi-variate process that recognises minority values, and thus demands that we have processes for values discovery. In Chapter 3 we discussed narrative rationality proposed by (among others) Brown (1990) and Habermas (1984). In essence, a rational process would build upon evidence *and* values through using this approach to offer a practical way forward that is ethically vigorous and practically robust.

Engaging all stakeholders

A good resource-allocation system will engage those most affected as far as that is possible. A robust process will incorporate one or more ways in which the public, patients and other stakeholders (GPs and the primary care team; secondary care providers; the local authorities; third-sector organisations) can be involved appropriately. Good public engagement is essential and must involve representatives of minority groups including Black and minority ethnic communities, health inequalities, particularly members of minority communities, refugees and asylum seekers, older people and those with specific needs that have often not been recognised.

Many attempts have been made during the last 20 years, especially since the advent of the internal market in the NHS (Daykin *et al.*, 2007; Honigsbaum *et al.*, 1995; Mullen and Spurgeon, 2000). These have included the following.

- Focus groups and other similar mechanisms of direct patient and stakeholder engagement, especially with minority communities (for illustration: Dolan *et al.*, 1999; Kitzinger, 1995; Robinson, 1999; Schultz and Angermeyer, 2003).
- Participant consensus conferences with a range of stakeholders to address marginal investment decisions or achieve consensus on treatment protocols (see, for example, Bero *et al.*, 1998; Curtis *et al.*, 2001; Einsiedel and Eastlick, 2000).
- Citizens Juries over two or three days, often also looking at marginal decision lists (see, for example, the DIY Citizens Jury, 2003; Institute of Public Policy and Research (IPPR); Delap, 1998; Gooberman-Hill and Calnan, 2008).
- Surveys of patients and the public, on (a) specific resource-allocation options, and (b) on the principles and criteria for making resource-allocation decisions, and (c) on the quality of care (for example, Roberts, 2001; Jenkinson *et al.*, 2002; Coulter, 2006).

The lessons from these experiments are somewhat daunting: it is very difficult to engage many stakeholders in the process because of complexity, cost, community interest, and other factors, but at the same time not to do so can lead to (small 'p') political problems that render ineffective any decisions taken. The tendency to pragmatism and special pleading will always be there. Achieving a process that delivers implementable decisions that can shift significant levels of resources will remain a real and difficult challenge.

Practical procedures for resource allocation

Many differing systems have been tried, especially for limited list resource-allocation processes. Mostly they have *not* been used to undertake zero-based budgeting processes, although these have been tried in the Netherlands and in New Zealand particularly. The 'necessary care' or 'basic package' of ideas that emerged for these countries may prove helpful. Mechanisms of priority-setting can be divided into those that use a limited list, those that use a multi-criteria process, and those such as the State of Oregon in the USA that have tried to create a comprehensive system for deciding on the best use of all the state and federal healthcare resources. It may be worth noting that many local authority systems do not try to be fully comprehensive, or at least they do not attempt to satisfy all demands made upon them. This is a reflection of the huge pressures on local authorities to manage many competing social care needs. Many have developed quite sophisticated systems of need determination which will come under severe strain during the next three or four years and will lead to further debate with the NHS on what will be funded.

Those systems, such as that developed in the South Central Region, tend to focus on single point interventions (a drug, device or procedure) for a specific indication. Topics come mainly from horizon scanning or from 'noise in the system' which means that they are often 'marginal' in terms of overall commissioning. Each topic is considered on its own: the decision-making is of the 'yes/no' variety rather than relative priority 'A or B or C, etc.', which means in turn that the question of affordability is not taken into account. The process does not weigh one investment against other possible investments/disinvestments that do not fit the evaluative framework and it is not always clear how 'priorities decisions' fit in the overall commissioning process.

An enhancement of this model provides a comparison of marginal investment possibilities. This has a recognised methodology which is useful in prioritising (marginal) investment, offers an 'objective' examination of the outcomes or benefits, enables decision-making to be more structured and explicit, and provides an audit trail for future reference. Each of these procedures has the advantage of flexibility, and helps to draw together colleagues from various professional backgrounds and achieved a level of consensus between competing professional opinions.

The perceived weakness of any marginal list system is that it needs sufficient background information, and requires careful selection of the right mix of people to reduce risks of bias. This suggests that the basic process is not sufficiently objective. The procedure demands adequate guidance on how to interpret each of the factors on which contender services are scored, and requires adequate preparation time to ensure all of the information which is being prioritised can be absorbed, and generates an occasional and natural tendency for some representatives to stress the importance of initiatives in which they have a degree of ownership or responsibility. The present process ranks on cost, once it is decided a procedure is worth funding, rather than on cost–benefit. Cost–benefit or cost–utility would help to identify where even low-cost and lower-priority interventions might nonetheless be worth doing because of the health gain achieved (Heginbotham et al., 1992).

The London School of Economics (LSE)[4] has developed what they term a 'Decision Conference', an extended meeting over two or three days in which the necessary information on alternative interventions and allocative opportunities is debated. The process (e.g. in Sheffield and the Isle of Wight) has focused on strategic interventions in specific care groups or programme budget categories. An emphasis is placed on the interplay of improving the health of the population (adding life to years, and years to life), reducing health inequalities,

---

[4] Professor Gwyn Bevan and colleagues, especially Dr Mara Airoldi. See the reference list.

improving the overall quality of care, and these are linked with feasibility and value for money.

Critical elements of the process are a focus on multi-criteria decision analysis within a CEA framework where the conference participants consider the health benefit generated per person, and the health benefits to differing population groups, from a number of differing interventions. This incorporates visual aids which are considered crucial to meaningful engagement, including a way combining clinical and epidemiological evidence, and exploring the value of interventions. The decision conference, and the process leading to it, is claimed to be a good way of engaging all stakeholders in debate, and overall it encourages engagement, systematic process and provides an audit trail. This has the advantage of enabling values, and the differences of values to be addressed, and offers sufficient time, albeit in a one-off conference for V-BC to be tested (see references, including Airoldi and Morton, 2009 and Airoldi et al., 2009).

One well-designed comprehensive priority setting scheme that uses multi-criteria decision analysis (MCDA), builds on accountability for reasonableness, and creates what its authors call a 'value matrix' as a core component of the process (Goetghebeur et al., 2008). The values matrix (VM) does not draw on individual or population values, but rather is a complex approach to assessing evidence and uses weights to give greater assurance and credibility to the determination of the correct intervention to use. The MCDA VM matrix does not include values that cannot be 'readily incorporated' and were set aside as 'extrinsic' values for consideration on a jurisdictional or case-by-case basis. These values included those of 'equity, historical context, stakeholder pressure, population priorities and access, and the ability of the health care system to make use of the intervention'. In other words, that is all those values that V-BP wants to make central to the debate. Using the term 'values matrix' may thus cause some confusion for V-BP as it is in essence a different process. Nonetheless, the EVIDEM framework (Goetghebeur, et al., 2008) is a well-designed approach that uses a structured, evidence-based approach to decide the best treatment to use for a specific condition.

A possibly better system is to use PBMA selectively alongside the careful construction of the problem. 'Programme budgeting' is a technique for describing where the money in a local health system, such as a PCT, has been deployed, broken down into manageable and meaningful programmes related to objectives, with the intention of tracking and influencing future deployment of programme resources (Brambleby et al., 2010). PBMA has two core features: first, there is no absolute right answer, but the analysis will raise more questions; and, second, looking at all programme categories and making a comparative assessment provides an opportunity to consider one programme in the context of all others. In values terms these features suggest maximising horizontal equity. In other words, PBMA levels the playing field and ensures all relevant information is included. PBMA simply takes what we know and makes it available in a way that encourages comparisons.

The comparison will suggest things that can be done differently. If a CCG (or PCT) with similar demographic numbers to your own is doing much better, either on cost or outcome or some other factor, this will offer suggestions for the way you can change your allocation to obtain an improvement. One CCG may be obtaining a good quality of care at median cost; this suggests that the high costs for the same quality in the second CCG may be amenable to improvement, but it will require careful analysis of the way that the first CCG has achieved the result. It may be spurious – that is always possible – or an artefact of the way that the data are collected; more likely, there will be particular ways in which the provider offers care that can be copied. (For a full discussion please see the analysis in Brambleby et al., 2010.)

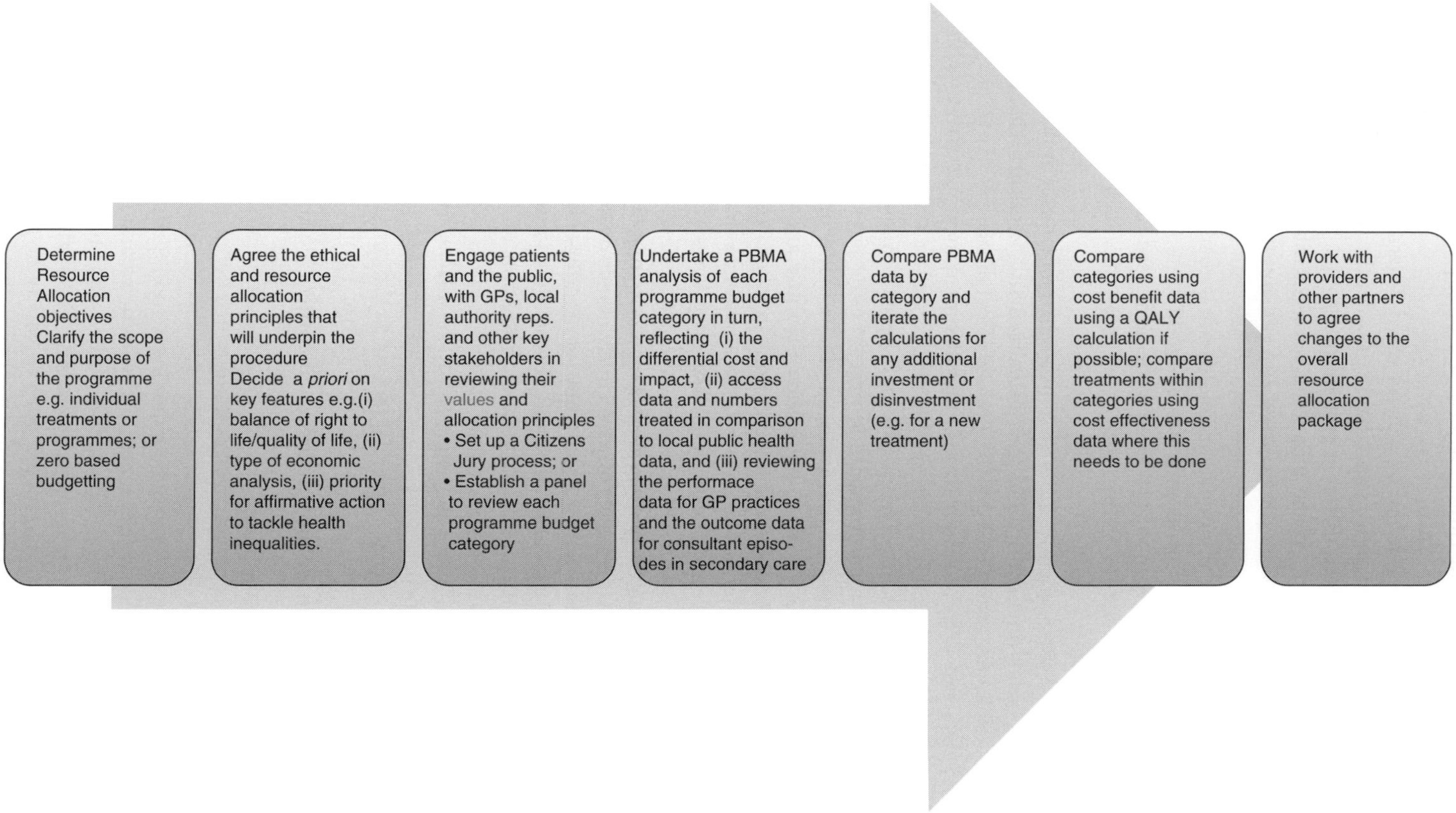

Figure 8.1 One approach to the priority-setting process.

Determine Resource Allocation objectives
Clarify the scope and purpose of the programme e.g. individual treatments or programmes; or zero based budgetting

Agree the ethical and resource allocation principles that will underpin the procedure
Decide a *priori* on key features e.g.(i) balance of right to life/quality of life, (ii) type of economic analysis, (iii) priority for affirmative action to tackle health inequalities.

Engage patients and the public, with GPs, local authority reps. and other key stakeholders in reviewing their values and allocation principles
• Set up a Citizens Jury process; or
• Establish a panel to review each programme budget category

Undertake a PBMA analysis of each programme budget category in turn, reflecting (i) the differential cost and impact, (ii) access data and numbers treated in comparison to local public health data, and (iii) reviewing the performace data for GP practices and the outcome data for consultant episodes in secondary care

Compare PBMA data by category and iterate the calculations for any additional investment or disinvestment (e.g. for a new treatment)

Compare categories using cost benefit data using a QALY calculation if possible; compare treatments within categories using cost effectiveness data where this needs to be done

Work with providers and other partners to agree changes to the overall resource allocation package

The marginal analysis calculations consider the cost of improving, or the cost savings of reducing, levels and/or quality of care. Margins are not necessarily small, but can be a large proportion of the baseline costs. By choosing the topic carefully, PBMA allows calculations of marginal net benefit from marginal investment decisions. PBMA will assist with making zero based-budgeting decisions if a CCG or other commissioner wishes to recalculate each programme or sub-programme against what we know about each clinical area. PBMA can be used as part of a programme, such as that shown below which attempts to make overall priority setting decisions.

Finally it is worth noting the results of the Oregon approach to seeking a comprehensive package of care that would be acceptable to the community (Honigsbaum, 1993). In 1989, Oregon, largely on the stimulus of one man, John Kitzhaber, decided to try to create a prioritised list of treatments that would be on offer to anyone to the extent the State and Federal funds would allow. In 1991, following a long period of preparation and consultation, Oregon had, through a complex process of caucuses and community meetings, ranked 700 services and agreed through the State legislature that it would be able to fund 587 of the 700 subject to Federal government approval (Oregon, 1991).

What is especially interesting for our purposes is the public values listed according to the frequency with which they were expressed at community meetings throughout Oregon (Honigsbaum, 1993, table 2, p. 24). These were grouped into three clusters: value to society, such as impact on society and personal responsibility; value to the individual, such as ability to function, or personal choice; and essential to basic care. Many of the values overlapped all three sections, including prevention, cost-effectiveness and quality of life. If done now, rather than 20 years ago, we may find a different result. However, what made Oregon so exceptional and distinctive was the determination to develop a public-funding mechanism that would benefit everyone, even though certain condition–treatment pairs would not be funded publicly for anyone.

The most useful processes drawn from these developments can be summarised in Figure 8.1 that brings together the differing elements. While this is comprehensive, and thus both extensive and time-consuming, if done correctly it will ensure the values of patients and service users are fully involved in the determination of the best balance of services to meet.

Conclusion

There are many ways to do priority-setting and resource allocation. The main lesson from this chapter is the importance of attention to balancing ethical principles and values-based statements about both the aims and objectives, and the processes of systematic examination of options. Too many priority-setting processes cut corners. Focusing on the four levels of the process described will ensure that all those involved will have an opportunity to influence (and be influenced by) the process.

Chapter 9

Outcomes-led commissioning

Developing a stronger focus on outcomes in health and social care has been an objective of the Department of Health and various institutions and academic bodies for at least the last 20 years. This quest for an effective outcome-based approach to commissioning and providing services was underlined again by the White Paper, *Equity and Excellence: Liberating the NHS* (Department of Health, 2010a) and associated working papers, notably the consultation on outcomes led commissioning, the *NHS Outcomes Framework 2011–12* (Department of Health, 2011c), and the consultation paper *Healthy Lives, Healthy People: transparency in outcomes* (Department of Health, 2011a, 2011b).

While an emphasis on outcomes is both timely and welcome the consultation papers have demonstrated once again the difficulties associated with identifying outcomes that are sufficiently robust to be used as contract currency. We take as axiomatic that a greater emphasis on outcomes is desirable and achievable, but recognise that implementing a truly outcomes focused approach will be enormously difficult for a number of reasons.

In a seminal paper, Donabedian (1988) demonstrated that quality in health care requires a proper integration of structural features (such as input resources and outputs achieved), processes related to offering care, and the outcomes of that care. He emphasised the importance of balance: every outcome has some form of supporting process which in turn requires a set of inputs. Focusing on outcomes to the detriment of inputs will not achieve the goal of improving outcomes; conversely placing undue weight on structural features (inputs or outputs) will not realise the best outcomes.

A brief example will suffice. Commissioning a health visitor service by the number of health visitor contacts with service users (an input factor) will not provide any information about the outcomes of those visits (the 'so what?' question); but commissioning using only a (relatively broad) outcome objective such as 'improved maternal and child relationship', however appropriate, provides no (or very little) information on the number of interventions that are likely to be required, nor it might be worth noting does it deal with the moral hazard associated with open-ended outcome objective where the use of resources is left entirely to the provider.

A renewed emphasis on outcomes often appears at times of austerity. For those who see the 'outcomes turn' as overdue, the emphasis is welcome; for others it might look like a not-too-sophisticated way to reduce cost and place the responsibility on providers to justify their funding against the outcomes they achieve. If outcomes were easy to define and measure this would be sensible; if that was true, an outcomes-led service would have been developed a long time ago. Unfortunately, outcomes are difficult to define, especially outcomes for the individual or group, and even more difficult to measure. It is little wonder that planners and politicians have defaulted to *output* measures as simpler to specify and easier to measure.

Outcomes can be described in many ways: for joint strategic needs assessment four levels were suggested (Department of Health, 2007) which we have used for the basic model of values-based commissioning: high-level outcomes (e.g. NHS or country-wide); second level – designed with communities in a locality or region as a way of expressing their involvement and expectation of change; third level – for groups of people with similar needs or common interests; and fourth level – outcomes for individuals especially those for whom a package of care can be designed. Alternatively, we can think about three groups of outcomes: individual outcomes, service outcomes and strategic outcomes (North West Roadmap).

Putting these together demonstrates the importance of a comprehensive approach to individual and service outcomes within a framework that recognises the inter-relationship of strategic decisions, service development and individual usage (see Table 9.1).

The NHS Outcomes Framework 2011–12 is designed to provide a national overview of how well the NHS is performing, provide an accountability mechanism to the Secretary of State, and act as a catalyst for driving quality improvement. Understandably this places an accent on high-level indicators for a programme of tackling health inequalities, reducing mortality and improving life expectancy. Nationally these indicators will provide an overview of population health, but they will not ensure that PCTs, CCGs and local authorities develop outcome targets that can be included meaningfully in provider contracts. As we move further towards competitive markets in health and social care (however slowly or quickly), whatever outcomes currency is used must be carefully defined, robust and enforceable.

Effective outcomes-led commissioning demands three interlocking sets of factors:

- outcome objectives that describe what the service is trying to achieve (the health and well-being objectives, containing a range of community and group values);
- outcome objectives that follow from the values of patients and service users; and
- a minimum set of features that enable the desired outcomes to be specified and used as a currency.

Table 9.1 Four-level population perspective and strategic, service and individual outcomes.

	Strategic outcomes	Service outcomes	Individual outcomes
High level	Accountability mechanism for quality improvement and health inequalities; mostly output or well-being measures	NAO, CQC and Monitor report on overall performance	Individual outliers reported by CQC
Community	NCB PCT Clusters and senates review outcomes for communities	CQC and Monitor review individual Trust performance	Locality arrangements offer high-quality care for individuals and groups with similar conditions
Group	Clinical Tsars report on specific condition–treatment arrangements	LA Scrutiny panels; HealthWatch	
Individual	Failures to meet basic care for individuals	Service arrangements that meet individual need	Outcomes for individuals are reported and investigated as required

Aggregating outcomes at individual level may tell us something about the impact on the group, or the local community. Unfortunately, most individual outcome measures do not aggregate readily – for example, pain or mobility before and after hip replacement. At a national level, statistically we may be able to say two things. First, that there were X% successful hip replacements, essentially an *output* rather than an outcome measure; second, something on general well-being improvement. Many of the proposed outcome indicators will be based on validated health and well-being instruments (such as EQ-5D), but adaptation effects[1] may undermine their value. Where these have the power to demonstrate that overall health status is improving or health inequalities are reducing they will be useful. However, by and large, these are service or strategic outcomes and do not relate *directly* to patients' experience of the NHS or the treatment they have received.

Dressing up output measures as outcomes does a disservice to the quest for effective outcome measures, and discourages commissioners from looking for new measures directly relevant and appropriate to service users and communities. Designing outcomes is hard. To be useable, outcomes must have all the following features to a sufficient degree: relevance to the care objective, directly measureable at reasonable cost and free from context and adaptation effects, causally associated with the intervention, comprehensive in covering all necessary aspects of the intervention, ideally capable of aggregation (at least to the group), and universal (i.e. to all those requiring that particular intervention). The latter does not preclude the need to ensure services are culturally relevant and meet the needs of minority groups in appropriate ways; and the value of 'proportionate universalism' (Marmot, 2010) in preventive and health promoting services should not be underestimated.

All these features are more or less complex amalgams of differing elements. An understanding of the relevance of an outcome feature, for example, demands an understanding of the context in which the individual requires the intervention, attention to personal characteristics, prior health states and co-morbidities, and the types of utility or well-being derived from the intervention. Some health care can be *relatively* straightforward from an outcome perspective (orthopaedic surgery) and some is not (long-term neurological conditions). Devising measures that are simple to understand and have performance management credibility (and leverage value) while taking into account the patients' complex responses to an intervention is challenging (Forder *et al.*, 2007). Measurement must be unbiased, scalable, free from confounders – all the requirements of good epidemiological research turned into robust, frequently used instruments.

Despite these headaches, commissioning for outcomes offers a step change towards services that are more attentive to the patient and service user. Personalisation of health and social care budgets (with or without direct payments) with an emphasis on clinically led commissioning within primary and community care requires a more nuanced understanding of what the patient or service user needs, the choices that service users make and the reasons for those choices, what constitutes a good outcome, and how that can be catalysed in clinically and cost-effective ways.

But there is a paradox. We need outcome data most in those areas where it is especially difficult to obtain: for complex long-term conditions; for the benefits of social care community interventions; for reduction in health inequalities and the results of affirmative action

---

[1] Adaptation effects are where the outcome effect attenuates or changes over time in a way that is unrelated to the intervention as the service user gets used to the improvement or deterioration in his or her condition.

to ameliorate 'prior discriminations'. High-level indicators will provide one part of the picture; the other part can only come from more investment in locally relevant, robust outcome measure that CCGs and local authorities can use to hold providers to account.

The process of tackling outcome measures is via a number of specific mechanisms within health and social care: QOF, QIPP and CQUIN within the NHS; personalisation and individual budgets in social care. The Quality and Outcomes Framework (QOF) is more concerned in practice with outputs than outcomes; QIPP is the programme on Quality, Innovation, Productivity and Prevention, which we have seen above; and Commissioning for Quality and Innovation (CQUIN) is the formal mechanism for promoting quality developments.

The QOF is a voluntary annual reward and incentive programme for all GP surgeries in England that describes practice achievement results. It is not concerned with performance management but with resourcing and then rewarding good practice. It contains four main components, known as domains: clinical, organisational, patient experience and additional services domains. Each domain consists of a set of achievement measures, known as indicators, against which practices score points according to their level of achievement. In the 2009/10 exercise QOF measured achievement against each indicator, up to a maximum of 1000 points. Although the four domains cover the main areas of practice, they do so from the perspective of financial reward for what is done – the higher the score, the higher the financial reward for the practice. While it might be thought that the domains would drive a values-based approach, in practice it offers an indication of the overall achievement of a surgery based on what they do rather than the way they do it (http://www.qof.ic.nhs.uk/). An online database provides easy access to comprehensive information on the pattern of common chronic diseases such as asthma, diabetes and coronary heart disease.[2]

While the QOF has had very little 'values' input, it assists practices to compare the delivery and quality of care currently provided against the achievements of previous years. Ultimately, the aim is to improve standards of care by assessing and benchmarking the quality of care patients receive. By collating world-leading intelligence on clinical areas, organisational, patient experience and additional services, GPs and other health professionals may have the basis for improvements in managing patient care, and particularly in developing a values-based commissioning process. Holding comparative information readily available about the quality of care and treatment will make it possible to use the data in focus groups, community and patient engagement processes and other mechanisms to involve patients more meaningfully. This will enable clinical commissioners, with patients and service users, to devise strategies for avoiding hospital admissions and thus develop alternative community services.

Recently, NICE has become involved in developing QOF indicators in addition to its work on quality standards. QOF indicators have not systematically taken cost-effectiveness into account and there is some evidence that the QOF payments do not adequately reflect the health benefit of the indicators. NICE has an acknowledged key strength in its robust processes for assessing clinical and cost effectiveness for use in the NHS. In addition, NICE has a Patient and Public Involvement Programme that encourages patients to engage in the process. This asks patients and the public to offer suggestions on the concept, definition and clarity of the quality standard, how appropriate the statements of quality

---

[2] Data for QOF is collected from over 8000 GP practices with over 54 million registered patients in England.

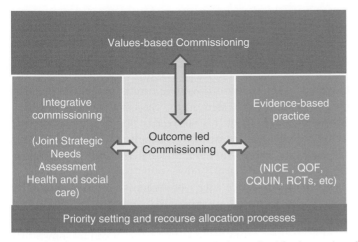

Figure 9.1 Values-based commissioning is at the heart of and fundamental to effective outcomes-led commissioning.

are, and whether the quality statements are measurable. In particular, NICE is concerned about whether the quality statements adequately cover the three dimensions of quality: safety, effectiveness and experience; how much a high-quality service could reasonably be expected to achieve; and whether the quality standards could be changed to better promote equity. This latter point covers access to high-quality services relating to age, disability, gender, gender identity, ethnicity, religion and belief, sexual orientation or socio-economic status.

Outcome-led commissioning is one strand of values-based commissioning (Figure 9.1), the others being integrative approaches, evidence-based practice, tied together by appropriate priority-setting and resource-allocation processes.

Any commissioning situation demands that we know what we are commissioning, and commissioning for outcomes demands clarity about aims and objectives, set by patients and service users with commissioning staff and provider clinicians. Commissioning for outcomes thus draws on values explicitly.

Social care outcomes

These outcomes can be considered in a number of theoretical ways, all of which demonstrate the complexity of the outcome and the problems of measurement (Forder *et al.*, 2007). There are seven models that are worth exploring a little:[3]

- welfare models,
- mandated welfare approaches,
- hedonic (happiness)-based systems,
- eudaimonic (flourishing)-based systems,

---

[3] This section draws on Forder *et al.* but in a substantially amended way. For a detailed and fuller discussion of these matters, see Forder *et al.* (2007).

- capabilities approach,
- life quality (QALY-based), and
- capacity to benefit.

The welfare model is closest to the values-based practice proposals that we are considering. Welfare systems should be based on individual assessments of health and well-being generated by an intervention, which in turn is predicated on the choices they make (or have made for them). However, the disadvantage is that it is not readily possible to measure the utility of an intervention directly, certainly not frequently or cheaply, and because patients and service users do not *in the main* pay directly for care, making cost–utility calculations becomes very difficult.

Welfare economics also suggest that a service user's preferences (choices) should be ordered, connected and transitive. In other words there should be a consistent list of the most desired to the least desired. This means that the person chooses the alternative that is most preferred over all others. The connectedness assumption requires that it can be shown that for each pair of alternatives either one is preferred to the other or the person is indifferent between them; and the transitive assumption says that if x is indifferent to y, and y is indifferent to z, then x is indifferent to z. This does not always hold, especially in political choices and we have to be careful about the context of use (Arrow, 1984, pp. 60–62). One of the challenges with welfare models is to develop a social outcome from collated individual outcomes.

In 'mandated' welfare models the NHS or a local authority dictates which outcomes are most important. Indeed, this is the present process whereby the NHS has decided on those outcomes that are to be measured. These of course may be helpful, or they may simply be the wrong choice! The critical issues raised by this approach are concerned with the impact on health and well-being of the policy selections. For example, if the NHS mandates a particular wheelchair to be used by all service users, it may impact on services as they will be able to plan for its use, but it may not be the most cost-effective.

In hedonic (or happiness)-based systems, the primary aim is to measure what makes people 'happy', usually although not exclusively by measuring the money value that individuals place on 'happiness'. Clearly, happiness is a pretty slippery and multi-faceted concept and not one that makes itself readily available to measure. However, the big problem is 'adaptation'. Over time people adapt to different health states or social situations. An able-bodied person might say that she would be deeply distressed if she became disabled; but when this happens the person in question may consider themselves fortunate, adapt to the circumstances and find a new way to lead a fulfilled life. That is not to underestimate the sometimes highly undesirable effects, but to recognise a truth – that people learn to live with many adversities. Love, relationships, fulfilment, academic achievement, sport – all these and many more lead to 'happiness'.

Eudaimonic models, conversely, place an emphasis on 'flourishing' (Keyes, 2002) rather than simply 'happiness'. They offer a different and usually better model for what really matters to people and are the basis of many health and well-being interventions that seek to maximise overall utility rather than simply what makes a person 'happy'. The idea of flourishing is that our lives are predicated on a number of factors. We are all different, and have differing needs, wants, desires and aspirations. What matters to us is the extent to which we want to and are able to achieve our goals. In that sense this approach reflects the 'recovery' model in mental health. We seek to measure the extent to which the mental health service actively enables individuals to achieve their life goals, based on their values and the ability of the service to assist. Some aspects of eudaimonic systems are as difficult as hedonic systems to measure directly and it suffers from some similar problems.

In the capabilities approach we focus on an assessment of an individual's range of capabilities and their ability to function on a day-to-day basis as an outcome of the service. This is more readily measurable, especially (although it is of limited value) by a simple scale (yes–no; or perhaps a three- or five-point scale). The capabilities approach reflects the challenges that have been made to welfare economics during the last decade. Instead of measuring welfare as subjective well-being, we seek to improve the ability of individuals to undertake particular tasks and to manage their own lives within society.

Focusing on the quality of daily life is unashamedly concerned with overall quality of life described as a QALY, or possibly a DALY, approach. The outcome of a service is measured as far as possible by using a series of quality of life domains of which there are many in the literature, but all of which include the following in one way or another: life and quality of life, interpersonal relations, emotional health, social inclusion, personal development, physical well-being, self-determination, making a positive contribution, choice and control, material or economic well-being, freedom from discrimination, civil legal and human rights, and bodily integrity.

Capacity for benefit is also a reflection of values-based commissioning, as it has both welfare and mandated welfare elements and links closely with the personalisation agenda – what the person wants allied with what the NHS or government wants. Capacity for benefit is an aggregated sum, rather than an individual perspective, and measures the potential of the service to deliver well-being according to a set of service domains relevant to patients or to service users. This is closely related to the 'equal ability to benefit' arrangement that we saw in the chapter on priority setting. By first addressing the health and social care inequalities suffered by those subject to prior discrimination, we seek to offer a level playing field from which everyone can benefit as equally as possible (Sen, 2002).

Those models and systems that are concerned with functioning suffer from a problem of thresholds for intervention, and will require some tough decisions. We want to ensure everyone is above a minimum level of functioning, but the outcome gain for a person below the threshold may be less (and less cost-effective) than for someone above that threshold. We may therefore have to forgo maximising cost-effectiveness in order to maximise the benefit to the worst off.

Measuring outcomes is not easy, which is why it is not surprising that government has chosen indicators that are mostly outputs rather than outcome, except where these can be considered outcomes of the service, rather than outcomes for individuals or groups. The reason it is difficult is that in defining outcomes we need to take a view on:

- the definition of *value* in the context of health and/or social care services;
- metrics or indicators of how much services deliver value (and inter alia the extent that this is value as described by service users and how much it is value from a 'value-for-money' cost-effectiveness perspective, which we have seen can be misleading);
- the consistency of improvements in function. This is, of course, related to evidence (functions derive from disease not illness) and thus is not strictly 'evaluative';
- The relative weightings of the dimensions of the measures so as to design a single composite measure of 'value change' (ONS, 2010).

Nonetheless, the Measuring Outcomes for Public Service Users (MOPSU) project has shown fairly convincingly, using the newly developed Adult Social Care Outcomes Toolkit (ASCOT), that, for instance, 'care homes delivered substantial outcomes for residents, significantly improving their quality of life, but were better at delivering outcomes in more basic areas such as ensuring residents were clean and presentable than in areas such as giving residents control over their daily lives'. MOPSU (using ASCOT) also found that day care centres were effective especially where users attended more than 3 times a week; and there was no difference between care homes in different sectors, except that third-sector homes 'tended to have fewer needs'. Interestingly, 'control over daily life' was found to be the most important social care outcome – a value that must be considered carefully in values-based practice (ONS, 2010).[4]

One vision of social care outcomes contains a strongly worded values statement. The Vision for Adult Social Care (Department of Health, 2010c) is based on creating incentives for prevention, extending personal budgets, and using direct payments to improve access to respite care. These statements contain values that are many people would generally accept at first blush. Prevention (rather than treatment or cure) means reducing cost and placing responsibility elsewhere than on the NHS or social care authorities; personal budgets means giving patients and service users greater say over the way their money is spent, but at the same time controlling the amount of money they can spend; and placing an emphasis on respite care. But on second thoughts, what do these values produce? The report suggests that it is based on three values: freedom, fairness and responsibility.

Freedom is a contentious value. As Claudio says in *Measure for Measure*, my 'present restraint is the consequence of too much liberty'. On the one hand it means positive freedoms to use resources as you think fit within a collective system of interdependence; or it can mean freedom *from* the constraining hand of local government to buy your care in the new social market that will develop. Fairness could mean equal shares of society's resources, based on a Rawlsian liberal consensus, where any derogation from equality benefits the worst off in

---

[4] 'The Measuring Outcomes for Public Service Users (MOPSU) project was a three-year research project to develop new, and examine existing, measures of the outcomes of particular public services. The project was funded by HM Treasury (HMT) under the Invest to Save Budget (ISB) and led by the UK Centre for the Measurement of Government Activity (UKCeMGA) at the Office for National Statistics (ONS) in partnership with three partner organisations:

- the Personal Social Services Research Unit (PSSRU) at the University of Kent
- the National Institute of Economic and Social Research (NIESR)
- the National Council for Voluntary Organisations (NCVO)

The project consisted of three main work strands with the overall aim of:

- more efficient and effective commissioning and procurement of services, placing the issues of quality and value for money at the heart of the decision-making process
- encouraging the use of 'outcomes' measures to assess the impact of services on their users, across the spectrum of providers
- examining the extent to which the third sector is involved in public service delivery and helping to alleviate barriers to entry to third sector organisations'. (ONS at http://www.ons.gov.uk/about-statistics/methodology-and-quality/measuring-outcomes-for-public-service-users/index.html)

society (Rawls, 1999); or it could mean seeking a way to use minimum resources to develop a home care system, for example while paying informal carers (which in practice means mostly women) and the third sector to provide the bulk of care. Responsibility could mean reducing dependency on the state by lauding 'personal responsibility' and 'freeing' communities and individuals to offer support, or it could mean the state taking responsibility by offering to underwrite support services.

None of these opposites is the last word: there will be consensus and compromise. However, it demonstrates the importance of pursuing a values-based agenda, and ensuring that all values are included with factual debate to identify the best way to offer care and to ensure that the services provided are the ones that individuals want. As the government acknowledge personal budgets are not an end in themselves: 'our focus is not on the process but on the outcomes of greater choice, control and independence' (Anchor *et al.*, 2011).

By tackling co-production (see the Chapter 7), it should be possible to cultivate a values-based practice that improves health and social care outcomes. 'One of the central ideas underpinning personal health budgets is that individuals are more than their medical conditions. They may have needs but they also have strengths and talents to contribute to the partnership alongside professionals' (In Control, 2009). Engaging patients and service users as 'co-producers', and using personal health and social care budgets, entails a rejection of the traditional view of patients. Instead, 'patients and service users become part of formulating the problem, identifying potential solutions, establishing outcomes, service delivery and evaluating effectiveness' (In Control, 2009).

NHS outcomes framework

The published NHS outcomes framework sets out six principles that should inform the way that outcomes are judged (Department of Health, 2011c). These will promote accountability and transparency, be balanced, focus on what matters to patients and healthcare professionals, promote excellence and quality, and focus on outcomes the NHS can influence but working with other public services where required. They will also be internationally comparable and evolve over time.

These will be used as a benchmark for five domains, in three groups. Group 1 is concerned with effectiveness includes: preventing people from dying prematurely; enhancing quality of life for people with long-term conditions; and helping people recover from episodes of illness or following injury. Group 2 is concerned with ensuring people have a positive experience of care; and Group 3 is safety – treating and caring for people in a safe environment and protecting them from avoidable harm (see Figure 9.2).

The critical question we need to ask is: to what extent have patients or service users and their carers had an opportunity to shape these outcome goals, and to what extent will their values be considered in deciding on priorities? For example, what are the respective contributions of the NHS, social care, the third sector and communities to these outcome measures, and what will we do if their views disagree, as they are likely to do, especially for community-oriented services? Many of the outcome measures proposed are not outcomes for service users. The term 'outcome' has been used rather loosely in places as a proxy for 'true' outcomes, and thus as a proxy for the outcomes that flow from a proper consideration of values. Outcomes must be relevant, measureable, associative, comprehensive,

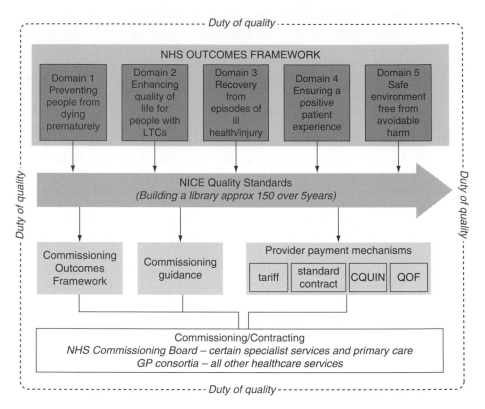

Figure 9.2 NHS Outcomes Framework – five domains.

summative and universal. And they must build on the values of the patients and service users.

End-of-life care

Let us consider end-of-life care. This has been identified by the Right Care group under the QIPP umbrella as an area that needs significant investment, of time and ideas, if not money. The End of Life Care workstream will focus on 'improving systems and practice for identifying people as they approach the end of life and planning their care' and it will place an emphasis on high-risk groups, such as those in residential and nursing homes. Working with NHS, social care and voluntary sector colleagues the workstream aims to:

- build a social movement for a good death,
- change national levers to support good end-of-life care,
- support the development of better intelligence about end-of-life care,
- help clinicians know when and how to start the conversation about end-of-life care,

- support systematic care planning, including Advance Care Planning, for people approaching the end of life, and

- identify and share successful good practice (http://www.dh.gov.uk/en/Healthcare/Qualityandproductivity/QIPPworkstreams/DH_115469).

The values that patients and service users bring to considering their own death will vary by age group and whether they have a terminal illness. In addition, planning end-of-life care is not concerned only with old age or cancer care. End of life can occur at any age; and the costs of end-of-life care are the largest proportion of lifetime health care costs. Between 60% and 70% of whole lifetime costs are usually expended in the last three months of any life, sometimes a higher percentage for younger patients. A young person with Acute Lymphoblastic Leukaemia, a road traffic accident victim who has significant acute trauma treatment but eventually dies, or a person with acute renal failure, all consume large costs that might be reduced (so that the money can be used more effectively for those that will live) through careful attention by clinicians to their prognosis.

What this turns on are our values about the futility, or at least the cost and benefits trade-off, of treatment – the forecast of when a person will not live whatever we may do. This challenges many 'sacred cows'. Who will say when my son or daughter or wife or partner will not be treated? On what basis? Not to have the debate leaves everyone open to the twin evils of (a) striving, sometimes 'officiously' to keep a patient alive, and (b) spending money abortively which could have been spent better. This is values-based practice at its sharpest. It demands values-based understanding of broad population (and political) perspectives, community views garnered by a range of alternate processes, group values for those with specific disorders (such as limiting long-standing disorders, or minority ethnic organisations, or older people), and individual understanding. Any commissioner has a tough task in finding a way to do this, and perhaps it is one of those subjects that needs a national, and rational, discussion. However, in practice these decisions are taken in every provider Trust every day, so a local commissioner response is not unreasonable.

A discussion of futility is rather easier in the UK than in the USA where it is infected by efforts to withdraw insurance funding, or to minimise its cost. Even in the UK, given the present government's attempts to encourage the market, there will be those who will obstruct a debate on the grounds that it is for the clinician and the patient alone to make the decision (Schneiderman, 2011). However, a discussion of futility (or latent futility) is overdue, not just for the very elderly or those with end-stage disease such as cancers, but for all those conditions that may affect people of any age. Some deny that futility should be discussed, but others disagree. 'Those who call for the abandonment of the idea of the concept [of futility] have no substitute to offer ... The common sense notion that a time does come for all of us when death exceeds our medical powers cannot be denied. This means that some operative way of making a decision when enough is enough is necessary' (Pellegrino, 2005).

A number of operational definitions have been proposed. First, values should trump; 'futility' applies when a treating clinician can do no more to meet the patient's wishes and goals. While it is essential that values are brought into the equation, especially to enable reflection on the evidence, it would be wrong to suggest that in all cases clinicians should accede to whatever the patient wants: especially as 'the physician does not owe the patient a miracle' (Schneiderman, 2011). The second definition is to make the definition of futility as narrow as possible, centred on physiological effects. This denies values completely and produces a narrow medical outcome based on 'fact' alone. Third, futility is defined as highly unlikely to prolong life. Here we must be careful. Prolonging life at all costs, when the body's organs are kept going by machine, is to be avoided if possible; but prolonging life has evident advantages. The critical factor is the degree to which the patient is able to use that life in some valued sense.

Shaping an operational definition for futility would benefit health care systems if it was possible to do so in a way that captured all the nuances and complexities of life. Of course it is true that for many years clinicians have been opposed to 'mercy killings', euthanasia, or for example pain relief that is given with just too much morphine. And there would have to be stringent safeguards. But all clinicians use medical futility at times. 'Do not resuscitate' directives are in use everywhere; nursing homes often allow patients to die at the home rather than forcing them go to the local hospital for heroic (and expensive) attempts to keep them alive for a few more days, or perhaps weeks. From a values-based practice perspective that is a challenge for commissioners – having a working definition that is used by clinicians at the correct time to alleviate suffering and to meet the values that the patient and his or her immediate carers will have discussed when the opportunity to do so was available.

The legal position is complex and any discussion of restricting treatments other than basic comforts and hydration could leave a hospital or nursing home open to being sued. The legal profession recognises that hospitals cannot continue to keep everyone alive who might

Non-Hodgkins Lymphoma: the example of Jaymee Bowen

Jaymee Bowen, or as she was known for quite a long time, Child B, became famous in the mid 1990s as a result of her father's attempts to force the NHS to pay for her treatment (Ham and Pickard, 2011). Briefly, Jaymee was diagnosed in 1990 at the age of six with non-Hodgkin's lymphoma, and was treated at Addenbrookes Hospital in Cambridge. She became ill again in 1993 with a second malignancy, acute myeloid leukaemia, but went into remission following treatment. Nine months later her leukaemia returned. Her treating clinicians all agreed that the chance of success of further treatment was approximately 1% (a 10% chance of remission following chemotherapy and a 10% chance the bone marrow transplant would be successful). The clinicians felt that the pain and discomfort together with the low chance of success meant that palliative care was in Jaymee's best interests.

At this point her father obtained a much better prognosis from clinicians in the USA although the UK clinicians stuck to their assessment. He obtained a referral to a doctor at the Hammersmith Hospital and asked the health authority to pay. The Medical Director refused. At this point one of the clinicians suggested a referral to the private sector and Jaymee commenced chemotherapy at the Portland Hospital and went into remission. Subsequently, the father brought legal proceedings against the health authority, which was unsuccessful, although it brought the case to the attention of the press.

The clinician at the Portland Hospital then had to decide how to proceed. Following a chance meeting with other clinicians, he decided to undertake a programme of lymphocyte infusion rather than a second bone marrow transplant. The treatment ended in July 1995. The health authority took over her treatment costs and the ban on reporting was lifted. Subsequently, however, Jaymee became ill again and this time the complications led to death in May 1996.

It is worth recognising the different values that were felt acutely: the agony of the father in contemplating losing his daughter; Jaymee's feelings of resignation at the endless and painful treatment; the clinicians' feelings about the treatment, some of which (notably the final lymphocyte infusion) were innovative and their effects in children, at that time, unknown; and the health authority's attitude to funding care that they considered was not beneficial. Eventually the treatment was stopped by Jaymee, who at the age of 11 made clear that she did not wish to have any further active treatment. The clash of values was intense.

One of the recommendations in Ham and Pickard is: health authorities should 'discuss and agree a set of values to guide decision making, building on the values laid down by Ministers, and involving other agencies such as NHS Trusts. This includes debating what those values mean and testing them in both hypothetical and actual cases' (Ham and Pickard, 2011, p. 89). While this goes some way to tackling the problem it does not go far enough. Although Ham and Pickard recommend clarity about consent for children and the availability of independent advice and counselling, they do not suggest that the values of the patient(s) (in this case, the father and Jaymee herself) should be made explicit and discussed as part of the decision-making process, especially where the treatment is likely to continue for some years and be very debilitating. That remains a challenge for commissioners to address.

want it, and that if we are to live within our increasingly scarce resources would it not be better to have the debate – facts *and* values – so that the resources saved could be used for those who would benefit, rather than those who would not.

Let us consider finally in this chapter an example of a patient where some of these considerations came into play in end-of-life treatment.

Conclusion

Defining outcomes is fraught with problems, especially if they are to be used for contractual purposes. While the NHS and local authorities might be prepared to operate to broad determinants without robust metrics, the private sector will not do so. Any contractual term will need to be sound, measureable and robust. Even the work on social care outcomes has not developed to the point that one could fine a provider for not meeting the outcome standards. Much of the government's approach is in practice to describe outputs, or at best outcomes for the service (which look remarkably like outputs). More importantly, determining outcomes is value-laden, both in their description and measurement. As we noted above, outcomes are an amalgam of values objectives. Only with a concerted attempt to understand patient and service-user values and create outcomes to match will outcome-led commissioning be fulfilled.

Market stimulation and market shaping

One of the most important aspects of commissioning, as we saw in Chapter 4, is the ability to develop or evolve a market for those elements that are not provided or are not provided well. Defining a 'market' demands that we consider basic aims and institutions. If the aim of the health service is to reduce cost, there will (probably) be an impact on quality. If the aim of the service is to ensure quality this will have an impact on costs. To make sense of this conundrum, the QIPP model (Department of Health, 2009) identified four key elements: quality, innovation, productivity and prevention. If we cut innovation (other than through 'lean' or similar methodologies) and prevention (other than for the most obvious elements of Health and Well-being) we can then concentrate on quality and productivity. Whether a quality and productivity strategy is better served by continued collective care, or by proportionate market development, will be discussed below.

Markets in health and social care, or at the very least the way they are described here, are fundamentally about values. We can see this in the way that markets have been discussed recently by the government, local authorities and health services. In describing market-led arrangements we note that patients and service users discuss the 'values' of those providing care and support; the way that priority setting processes place values centrally in making decisions about the availability of a treatment; or the emphasis of hospital Chief Executives on discharge criteria. Markets are a good example of values-in-action. Holding to the idea of NHS and social care as collective provision supported by a covenant between the government and people is an attractive idea; conversely markets are a way of achieving 'best value' through competition. Collective care supports equality; markets support innovation.

Values, as we shall see, are engaged seriously in developing market solutions. This is in part a result of quite grotesque market failure which has placed large numbers of elderly and mentally handicapped individuals at risk, and in part a determination of the government to develop a 'market culture' within the NHS and social care without serious debate. Each of these has raised the public's fascination with the market and its operation, reflecting their concerns, their overall lack of information, and the known extent of the market once it is described. 'Market stimulation', however, is a value in itself. Having a range of providers offers a range of quality, price and specification that suggests choice and opportunity. Of course, whether these can be afforded remains uncertain.

The design of a market system depends on a number of factors and this encourages a debate about the values that apply. The first of these is the right of a patient to choose linked with a series of principles for competition, either a regulatory framework or some form of statutory guidance. In the Principles and Rules of Cooperation and Competition (PRCC) the

Department of Health has developed as a framework for the healthcare system. Choice is a critical element and it is one where differing values and needs find ready expression. Choice is thus a simple yet powerful indicator of the way that any health system operates. Does choice mean that we must offer alternatives to the NHS, or does choice operate at the edge of the system where those looking for health care fail to find it locally at a sufficient degree of quality? Does choice mean a minimum of redundancy, which either costs more or reduces quality?

The PRCC will be guaranteed by the Cooperation and Competition Panel that is soon to move into Monitor as a separate function, and will in the long term decide on the extent to which competition becomes an endemic feature of the health (and social care) system, or is a marginal development. In practice it is likely that competition will continue to develop over time and values-based practice will not hinder but rather help that development.

Choice and related aspects has been a feature of the NHS since it was created, but in the last few years has been elevated as a method of enabling patients to obtain care that is appropriate for them. Patients in England requiring routine elective care have been able to choose between the NHS and independent sector provision registered with the Care Quality Commission (CQC), has a PCT or nationally let contract and is willing to provide services at the NHS tariff. Some 15% of PCT expenditure is covered in this way and is expected to grow over time. However, some PCTs have been found to be excessively constraining choice and providers' ability to offer routine elective care, although this varies considerably. PCTs appear in some instances to be deliberately influencing GP referral decisions away from certain providers, although often for good reasons, such as helping the PCT to remain within budget. PCTs have a number of mechanisms for doing this including caps on the number of patients a provider can treat.

The CCP's approach to 'assessing restrictions' is to 'balance the costs to patients and taxpayers of a restriction against any benefits that arise from that restriction' (CCP, 2011, para. 11) Commissioners should use 'mechanisms that target overall demand' (CCP, 2011, para. 12) rather than explicit numbers by provider, as this would restrict choice. What do we consider as a component of the costs to patients of a restriction? It might be argued that the costs are not simply those financial costs that can be summed readily, but should include the role of values and value-costing. The values of patients and service users are rarely exclusively to have the elective procedure done as soon as possible. Often, a range of values will be engaged: the value of having a consultant and care team that is known and understood; the value of a GP–Consultant relationship; the value of a continuum of care between hospital and community services, especially if things go wrong; the value of having a local service rather than one at a distance; the negative-value of choice when the only reason for choice is that there is no choice; the values of 'integration'; and last but not least, the 'value' of the NHS as a worthwhile enterprise as part of the social contract.

The social contract is not an argument often run by those espousing markets. Government has sought to play down the importance of the NHS as a component of the post-war settlement, with the 1948 National Assistance Act, the NHS, the 1944 Education Act and the other elements of a social democratic ideal. Some markets are a good thing: where there is no present service or the NHS cannot afford to provide; some services, such as homeopathy that are highly tendentious; some services, including elective care, where the NHS has for whatever reason decided not to provide. However, for many services, Nye Bevan's stricture at the beginning of the NHS on 5 July 1948, that 'private charity can never be a substitute for social justice' rings as true now as it did then. Privatisation may solve a problem, although as we have seen, under-regulated care is no substitute.

The infrastructure for assisting choice is, as we saw in Chapter 1, largely mechanistic and evidence-based rather than values-based. Choose and Book, Payment by Results and NHS Choices all offer information but little opportunity to change the basic system of care. The Principles and Rules outlaw the restriction of choice without good reason, other than to create a market and allow other providers a free rein. Where alternative providers can offer a service is to minority groups especially Black and minority ethnic communities. Those groups and community organisations that wish to do so may be able to provide certain components of care that would either not be provided or demonstrate elements of discrimination. Commissioning actively with and on behalf of minority groups can assist in ensuring that the service is acceptable and that the groups themselves may be able to offer part or all of the care.

Market stimulation offers opportunities for minority providers to suggest care alternatives that are culturally relevant and appropriate or include specialised approaches that only the minority community provider will understand fully. Comprehensive market systems include private, independent, social enterprise and third-sector providers that not only offer choice but a range of culturally specific and values-based notions of what matters. Within certain quality constraints, some patients will want the most cost-effective, efficient and professional provider; others may want to know that the organisation is a non-profit body using all its resources to the benefit of patients.

Model markets

Once a health or social care system contains a range of choices (about the use of hospital or community services, or about provision of domiciliary care, or a specific service) other factors come into play. A 'model' market includes a number of features (in the main mostly related to social care, although the following paragraph applies just as much to the developing market place in health care) of which segmentation is most important. Segmentation can develop in a number of ways: through demand-side and supply-side conditions; geography (place-based services); economies of scale; and provider market niches – catering for specific, and often rare or expensive types of care. In addition, the type of market will be relevant (e.g. community, primary, acute, long-term, social care, domiciliary care, etc.); there will be barriers to entry and exit, and the symmetry or asymmetry of information will be important.

These features lead to widely differing market arrangements especially in social care, where service users have delegated individual budgets to buy a range of help and support. Markets then develop on the basis of the extent of choice offered which in turn is dependent on the numbers of providers, their rivalry and the ease of switching between them.

The final criterion is customer quality. Quality is both a prior determinant and an outcome of the service. In that sense it can be used to drive the features of a service or it can be the aim of the service – ex-ante or ex-post determination of its utility. If the quality is good then we can move on to consider other aspects of the service; or we aim to achieve a good quality by arranging the features of the service to achieve a high level of satisfaction with the service. 'Quality' is of course a value-driven term. 'Quality' derives from a number of significant features including the 'value' of the service offered – what the customer thinks of the 'value for money' of a service, which in turn derives from a cost–quality trade-off. Quality depends on a range of values, including the following (developed from QIPP Right Care, 2010).

Box 1. Quality and values (QIPP Right Care, 2010)

- Subjective evaluation of the quality of a service or a treatment provided. For a patient, clinical treatment will depend on many factors, but which of them are most important? Is it the bedside manner of the surgeon, or that the toilets are clean? If the patient has a professional background in medicine she will be more critical of the medical care than someone for whom it is an alien experience. Any subjective assessment takes all these features into account.

- Non-clinical quality. We know we cannot afford the ultimate quality for everyone, but we can (and should) ensure that at least the clinical quality remains as high as possible even if the non-clinical quality is less than excellent. Paradoxically non-clinical quality is the area of most peoples' expertise, whereas for many the level of clinical quality remains beyond their knowledge.

- Clinical quality. Clinical quality is the aspect of a service that most drives an individual assessment, but the features to include are contentious. The clinical quality of a medical or surgical procedure includes at least the following:

  - the level of clinical expertise of the nurses, the doctors, and other key clinicians, including their training, assessment, and on-going support;

  - decisions about the desirability or otherwise of the treatment, and whether or not this has been discussed between the patient and the clinical team;

  - clinical assessment or diagnosis and associated facts, such as the patient's condition, co-morbidities and lifestyle;

  - availability of the service or part of the service that is appropriate to the patients' needs (in other words, has the priority-setting and resource-allocation process ruled out part of the necessary care);

  - purchasing or allocation of drugs and medicines for the complete cycle of care required;

  - levels of care for a complete recovery based on the patients' own assessment of what a complete recovery means.

- Support from significant others. Some aspects of health and social care require support from informal carers, such as relatives, or volunteers, or other critical friends.

- Geographical provision, including travel time and convenience.

The quality debate is thus broad and deep, and defies easy answers. 'Quality' becomes a rather haphazard concept, given additional features when these are known or essential, or left undefined where this aids debate. And yet quality is the driving force. The present Department of Health policy on QIPP suggests that quality is given a leading aspect alongside innovation, productivity and prevention. In practice, of these elements, 'productivity' has the edge in deciding on the costs of services. And this is to be expected from the previous discussion. Innovation is an essential vehicle for change but cannot be delivered 'just like that'; 'prevention' is a critical aspect of care and support, and yet is overlooked except at the margins where it demonstrates a short-term payback, say over two or three years. The prevention agenda is important and becoming more so over time. However, there is a lot of reluctance within the NHS and social care, especially to spending money on weakly or non-evidenced-based, or long payback, programmes.

In trying to decide whether a 'market' will improve quality there is a real dilemma. Do we simply accept that some aspects of a market will by definition improve quality, or do we ask more searching questions? Will the private sector improve quality, as we have defined it above, or will it leave some patients to the mercy of the staff as we saw at Winterbourne View (see, for example, BBC news report, 1 June 2011), or to the mercy of the market at Southern Cross (http://www.guardian.co.uk/business/2011/jul/16/southern-cross-incurable-sick-business-model).

If these market arrangements did not work for patients, can we pose a viable market strategy, including the private sector, not-for-profit organisations or the third sector? The answer has to be 'yes', if only because local authorities place so many patients with private organisations. But for the future, so much will depend on company structures with significant controls that ensure viable and effective arrangements. Third-sector and community group programmes may be highly relevant to the market, but if they are to be included this means an open market system with a system of controls that ensure a range of opportunities and outcomes. What might this look like?

First, it requires a set of regulatory elements that place a premium on social enterprise and patient support; and, second, it demands that all companies work on a genuinely level playing field, in which the third sector or community group is treated no less, but no more, favourably than the private or statutory sector. Recognition of the importance of process and governance is needed in the special relationship with the third sector and community groups.

Developing a true 'market' in health and social care argues for a range of options including the opportunity for third-sector and community groups, especially but not exclusively for Black and minority ethnic organisations, to be involved in commissioning health and social care, and to be engaged as providers of significant albeit specialised forms of care. These latter include advocacy, citizens advice, and community services. Their involvement is predicated on a market arrangement that recognises their distinct contribution in the context of statutory or private provision. Undoubtedly much of this will be small-scale, but need not be, which poses a challenge to commissioners to reach out and engage these groups. (Chapter 6 discusses engagement mechanisms.)

If a third sector or community group is to apply to provide a service it will be essential for that group to identify a substantial range of values, from its view about the minority community that it represents to the importance of specialist therapy or treatment that it has inherited or developed. The group may have a very different values-based opinion about the nature and disability of its members compared to the commissioning group, and may have a robust opinion on the type of care that should be offered.

Segmentation of a market ensures that the needs of all groups in society, but especially minority groups (e.g. Black and minority ethnic elders) receive the right level of choice of provider. This is an area where values are especially prevalent. Minority groups may have rather different values and these will be evident when there is any discussion about the levels of care and those who might provide that care. Black groups may be in a better position to offer care that has the values of the community in mind.

Demand- and supply-side constraints determine what can and cannot be readily provided. For example, a demand-side constraint will be the extent to which patients may or may not be willing to switch between substitute services, such as between a coronary artery graft and watchful waiting. Supply-side requirements suggest that providers must be able to switch resources from one treatment modality to another as a result of choice or demand. An example might be of a provider geared to offer in-patient support for diabetes who recognises that the service may be more readily and more cheaply provided in the community.

A number of other criteria need to be considered at this point. Geography, market niches and competition all offer alternatives for patients. Geography is an important consideration in relation to differing aspects of illness: in some cases, a patient would not be prepared to travel for limited short-term 'every day' treatment, but a minority group member may be prepared to travel considerable differences for a culturally relevant solution. Similarly, a mentally ill person may be happy to travel quite a long way to obtain a treatment that is only provided by a small handful of providers. This may apply to market niches where a health care supplier makes a specific provision that is not generally available (but is not so expensive or specialist that it comes under one of the specialised commissioning arrangements). This will follow the same logic to that used for the determination of the type of care offered. As commissioners seek to detach health care from acute hospitals (except where quite appropriately the care requires in-patient support) there will be an expanding number of alternatives offered, either by the NHS, by private organisations or the third sector. The latter are in a good position to offer culturally relevant and appropriate forms of care.

Barriers to entry and exit from care are serious constraints on the development of alternative provision. Some types of care – hospital care, for example – have large entry and exit barriers, normally as a result of cost. Conversely, community alternatives have relatively low barriers to entry or exit and are much more flexible. We can see this (in Chapter 11) in Michael Porter's five forces. The way that substitutes are used is (in part) determined by the cost of substitution.

Economies of scale have a significant effect on the location and decentralisation of care. Some services may be better located for clinical, economic, workforce or population perspectives on a larger footprint in a way that achieves savings. Here we must recognise the values-based demands that minority groups (and not simply BME groups) may pose. There may be an economy of scale, but to what extent is that accepted by everyone, or indeed anyone? An individual or a group in society may agree that the overall level of care is achieved by sensible and contractually reasonable economies but may still not wish to be treated in that way. Their argument may be that the service is too distant, or insufficiently attuned to their culture, or has sexist or racist overtones.

Q4C: a model of markets in health and social care

The next four features (the Quality and four 'Cs' or Q4C model) are perhaps the most important for quality: overall quality in the market is dependent on choice, concentration, cooperation, and competition. Values-based practice is especially relevant in this area. The values espoused by clinicians, especially doctors, and those of nurses, psychologists, social workers, and other social care staff will vary noticeably, and they are likely to differ markedly from those of patients and the public. Let us consider the four 'Cs' in turn (Figure 10.1).

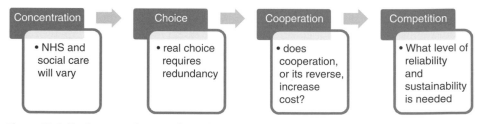

Figure 10.1 The four main elements of a market.

Concentration

Concentration is the degree to which provider activity is focused on a small number of providers. Let us consider the example of six providers of banking services. Although of similar size, five may be mainly commercial and only one predominantly retail. The 'concentration index' (Herfindahl–Hirschman Index)[1] will give a misleading impression: it will suggest that there is competition when in practice competition does not exist (Herfindahl Index; Hirschman, 1964; Wikipedia, 2011). In this case, customers of the retail bank may be affected as a result of the market dominance of this one firm; the market is not properly defined because cheque accounts are not a substitute for commercial or investment banking. To take another example, one cinema may have 90% of the market for attended films locally, but if cinemas compete with video hire shops, 'Love Film', or televised films, then people are less likely to be suffering due to market dominance. Another typical problem is geographical scope. For example, firms may have 20% market share each, but may occupy five areas of the country in which they are monopoly providers and thus do not compete against each other.

Interestingly, the average index for London PCTs is 4000 (Ernst and Young, 2011) and most probably higher outside the South East. Whether a patient or service user has choice will be dependent on the concentration levels for relevant providers. Concentration affects the market and thus customer choice simply by reflecting the number of providers available for the patient or service users needs – condition and treatment, social care opportunities and so forth.

Choice: patient and service-user options

The Department of Health states that it is committed to giving patients choice of treatment and provider wherever possible. Money will increasingly follow patients' choices and reward providers that offer high-quality services in response to patients' preferences. Monitor, the health regulator, will promote patient choice and competition for services on a level playing field and will have powers to address restrictions on competition where this acts against the public interest. The best NHS providers should thrive, as more patients choose to use them, and funding follows those patients. Competition and a national tariff will create strong incentives for other providers to improve. Those providing poorer quality or unresponsive or inefficient services will come under increasing pressure either to improve, sell out to an alternative provider, or close. Whether these options are ones that CCGs will wish to give early consideration is difficult to follow. However, there is no doubt that some of the CCGs will be faced early on with some very difficult examples. Of course 'having choice' is a value as is 'being able to choose'; but for the Department of Health it counts more as a proxy for competition than as a value for patients.

Monitor is currently the regulator for foundation trusts and already has the status of a non-departmental public body. Subject to discussion in parliament, the Department of Health was proposing to develop Monitor into an economic regulator for all providers, rather than establishing a new body to take on that job. Monitor's role as economic regulator was to ensure that the social market for provision of NHS services operates in the public interest by promoting patient choice and competition, where appropriate, and regulation of providers, where necessary. This will be in the context of making substantial savings by reducing bureaucracy and reviewing the Department's arm's-length bodies.

---

[1] The Herfindahl–Hirschman Index (HHI) ranges from 10,000 for a monopoly provider to 100 for a range of providers. The HHI is a measure of the size of firms in relation to the industry and an indicator of the amount of competition among them.

However, as we saw in Chapter 2, the role now given to Monitor is to protect and promote patients' interests and it will not be expected to 'promote' competition *as an end in itself*. Monitor will be limited to tackling specific abuses and unjustifiable restrictions that limit patients' interests, and the government has accepted that Monitor should not 'open up competition by ... allowing access to its facilities to another provider'. Whether this will have the effect desired by the Futures Forum is debatable, especially as Monitor will have powers concurrent with the Office for Fair Trading has to the EU to ensure competition rules are applied effectively. Consequently choice will remain and be imposed legislatively and through the NHS constitution.

Cooperation

The term 'cooperation' (or a lack of cooperation), sometimes referred to as 'switching', indicates the 'churn' in the market, the number of patients (or CCGs/PCTs/social care providers with changing patient/service user numbers) from one year, or monitoring period, to another. Often this cannot be detected directly, although in some cases CCGs/PCTs/ Health and Well-being Boards may identify the change in the form of contract amendments. CCGs/Health and Well-being Boards will have a difficult task in the first couple of years understanding the extent of cooperation where patients have an opportunity to change provider, although in most acute services the likelihood of major changes is small. What does matter, however, is whether quality is the driver, or whether the PCT (or in future the CCGs) and Health and Well-being Boards drive quality by forcing an anti-cooperative movement of patients or service users from one service to another. As provider competition increases, patients and service users will be able to shop around, increasing transaction costs, and potentially using more than one provider simultaneously for the same treatment.

Cooperation suggests two ways of thinking about commissioning: the ex-ante position, where quality is measured and mechanisms are arranged to force a change of provider(s); or an ex-post arrangement, where quality is achieved by setting the characteristics of the providers with a particular level of quality in mind.

Competition

Sometimes referred to as 'rivalry', this term refers to the competition between providers. This has some significance, as actual markets are characterised by real entry and exit. Indeed, over the previous two years or so we have seen a substantial increase in the number of firms going into administration, and some have not survived. In the community health and social care market there is every opportunity to develop new, cheaper or more appropriate care, especially from individual health and social care budgets controlled by service users, which will bring with it the likelihood of some market failures. Some of these failures are as a result of changes to the care provided; some are because the provider simply cannot cope with the change.

One of the present government's considerations has been the extent to which providers may 'cherry pick', leaving the NHS to deal with more difficult or expensive cases. This concern has been expressed vociferously by those worried about the NHS, and it has been accepted, albeit in a way that suggests the problem will be allowed to bite further along the track. Services will be covered by a system of prices that accurately reflect clinical complexity, *except where that is not practical*; and commissioners will be required to follow best value principles when tendering for non-tariff services rather than simply choosing the lowest price. These sentiments, drawn from a Department of Health document, sound as though the government has taken into account the calls from lobbies for controls on market stimulation. Yet in practice these are easy words and do not of themselves absolve the NHS or anyone else from the worst effects of the market.

The Department of Health goes on to say that 'we will outlaw any policy to increase the market share of any particular sector of the market'. What this means is open to question. The government has stated that Monitor will continue to pursue EU competition law, and to act in a sector-specific role; yet here it states rather boldly that we will outlaw *any* policy that seeks to increase market share. It suggests that the civil servants drafting the statement have taken to heart the views of those campaigning about the Bill and have accepted that '[w]hat matters is the quality of care not the ownership model'.

Of course, policy statements about the quality of care may well be developed to encourage a range of providers, and this will be helpful for those services that PCTs and CCGs believe can be improved through market testing. As the Government's Response to the Health Select Committee (2011), made clear, commissioners should not compete on price where there is no agreed tariff but on value, and seek to achieve value from the offerings of differing providers.

Managing the market

Once we have all four of these elements in place we can use the information realistically to develop a process of market stimulation and influence. At present the majority of services where markets are involved in social care especially for those requiring long-term support, or within services for people with mental disorder, and in learning difficulties, where there is a significant proportion of private provision. Many of these are quite local and agreeable to close involvement with the local health or social care authority, but some are both much less engaged and more competitive in their approach.

Let us take an example. Whether we consider quality as ex-ante or ex-post, we can see what the implications of values-based practice for market stimulation might be. If we consider the quality of existing services to be good then we need to look at concentration. If this is low there may be a good reason to change the way that services are provided. This will automatically improve choice, and then cooperation, and finally competition. If increasing concentration simply is not possible (or only at the margins) then choice will not be possible and alternative strategies may be required. On the other hand, if the quality is not good, whether there are a lot or a few providers, it may be necessary to encourage more providers, or to change the contract. In the former case cited here the concentration goes down (numbers of providers increases) and patients need to be encouraged to choose between them based on information offered by the CCG; if, conversely, the CCG decides to tender and to offer a single contract, choice becomes limited but at least, all being well, the quality of care improves.

So what is the extent of values-based practice in these cases? It will be clear that two aspects need to be considered. First is the attitude of patients or service users to quality; and second, to concentration. If these two are considered first, most other aspects fall into line. If concentration improves (i.e. goes down) then it is likely there will be greater cooperation (switching), and if that happens it will drive competition (rivalry). Quality considerations demand that the commissioner understands the nature of quality and the extent of agreement by the patient to the providers' quality criteria. For example, the commissioner may suggest that quality is dependent on cost. A cost–quality trade-off will have been the first thing the commissioner will have considered. However, what (s)he will probably not have considered is the attitude of the customer (patient or service user) to that trade-off. It is worth noting here that the government has said firmly that price competition will not be allowed. Price will be fixed (via Payment by Results) and competition will be on quality alone. This of course begs a number of questions, notably on the way quality is measured and compared.

Many FTs will have made decisions about the nature of quality without properly informing the service user. An example is provided by the closure of old-fashioned mental health services, resulting in long and rather bitter campaigns to keep the services open. The service users and their carers may lose the battle not because of the attitude of the provider, but because of the attitude of the commissioner, who either does not come to the aid of the service users, or expressly assisted the process by stating their preference for the alternative. As an aside, this approach of leaving services to the provider to sort out is both a real frustration for the provider, as well as guaranteeing cynicism about commissioning.

If commissioners do not engage in a discussion about the values of the service with users and carers, or do not engage with the community in a meaningful way, then the potential for values-based improvements is limited. What will happen is that the lack of a values-based understanding will have angered the service users such that they may take vengeance on the decision at some point, or the opportunities to find an a viable, reasonable and cost-effective alternative solution will be lost.

Market evolution

As we have seen, markets depend on four factors: sufficient providers with an interest in the service that you have in mind; patients or service users ready to choose between providers; customers (patients or service users) prepared to switch from one provider to another; and competition between providers for the business. This has been characterised in an influential and informative way by Michael Porter (*Competitive Strategy* followed by *Competitive Advantage*). In these books, Porter describes the market as five 'forces' operating either to achieve equilibrium or for one of the 'players' to dominate over time (Figure 10.2).

The five forces determine industry profitability because, 'they influence the prices, costs and . . . the elements of return on investment' (Porter, 1985). The strength of each of the five forces is a function of 'industry structure', which is relatively stable but can change over time. Unfortunately this model does not hold well for health care and a differing approach has been proposed recently. Value (not 'values') is, on this argument, the key. 'Value' will require a 'fundamental restructuring of the health care delivery'; Porter suggests that the central goal of health care is 'value for patients' and uses the full set of patient health outcomes and the total costs of care for the patient's condition.

This provides part, but only part, of the equation. Focusing on outcomes is, as we have seen, challenging, but patient outcomes are the necessary objective of values-based commissioning. By using all the values that patients bring it is possible to expand the 'value' description beyond 'value for money' to a wider conception of outcomes. Porter's solution is structural – to organise into integrated practice units around patients medical conditions. Drawing on US primary care physician practice he proposes moving to bundled prices for care cycles (i.e. equivalent to Payment by Results) and integrating care delivery across separate facilities. It is difficult to see how this would work in the UK without destroying primary care and clinician-led commissioning. Alternately, provider integration is needed

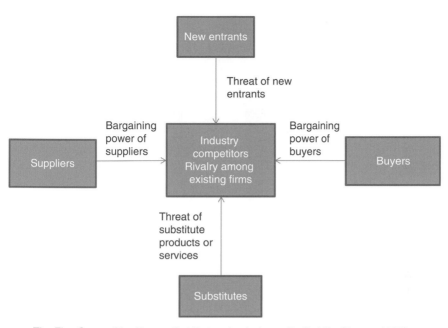

The Five Competitive Forces that Determine Industry Profitability (Porter, 1985)

Figure 10.2 Five competitive forces that determine industry profitability. Reproduced by permission of Prof. Michael Porter, Harvard University Press (Porter, 1985).

based on clinical groupings that bring together primary, community and acute services with clinical pathways acting as the glue for common patterns of care.

'Values', be they from professional staff, patients and service users and carers, or the public, can be the drive of any health system change. Drawing on values will ensure that the structure and processes of care are right as well as the outcomes, and using values-based practice will influence the solution proposed by Porter, or other commentators. In health care the systems are rather different, even allowing for private-sector involvement in the market. We can see in Figure 10.3 some of the implications and in Figure 10.4 we see the way that an integrated system might work.

The system may become complex, with a range of public and independent providers competing in the same place 'for the market'. This occurs now in social care for older people, in mental health, learning disability and a few other areas. Whether the costs are reasonable is a factor. It might be argued that the government's approach to markets and competition as exemplified by the CCP paper (2011) creates the environment for a more far reaching change towards individual practice units (IPUs), specialised primary care physicians, with a wide range of 'in the market' and 'for the market' opportunities. As these become established, commissioners will slowly change from being planners and purchasers of blocks of services for communities to insurers offering individualised medical and social care. This may seem like a good idea for those wanting long-term care (for example, diabetes or neurological problems) using an integrated health and social care budget, but if this becomes the norm, it may lead to the establishment of a social insurance model.

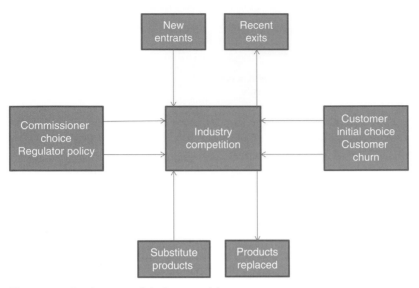

Figure 10.3 Developments of the Porter model.

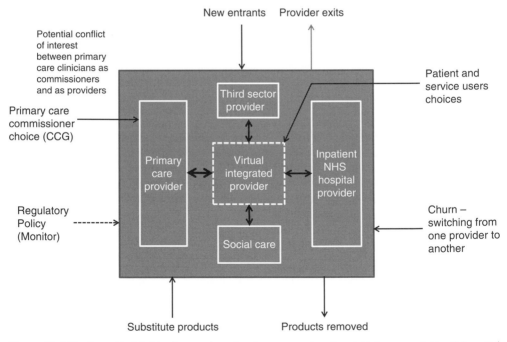

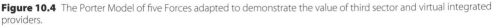

Figure 10.4 The Porter Model of five Forces adapted to demonstrate the value of third sector and virtual integrated providers.

Monitor's role

Monitor will carry out three core functions as economic regulator:

- promoting competition,
- regulating prices, and
- securing continuity of supply where there is no alternative provider(s).

Monitor will work with the NHS Commissioning Board to regulate prices for NHS services. Effective price regulation will support investment in NHS services by creating a more transparent and predictable system of reimbursement and strengthen incentives for providers to improve quality and efficiency.

Initially, Monitor's functions will apply to healthcare services, but provision will be made in the Health Bill to extend Monitor's functions to adult social care, subject to affirmative resolution in Parliament. Monitor's regulatory powers will apply equally to all providers of NHS services and organisations in the private and voluntary sector.

As in the current system, commissioners will retain responsibility for ensuring the continuity of service provision. Monitor will be able to identify services that require additional regulation and set conditions in providers' licences to protect the continuity of those services. Monitor will be able to require contributions to a risk-pooling system to ensure the continuity of services in the event of failure as well as being able to intervene directly in the event of failure, and trigger a special administration regime to secure continuity of supply.

The CQC currently registers providers of health and adult social care services to offer assurance that they meet essential levels of quality and safety and they will continue to exercise this role. Monitor, on the other hand, will license providers of NHS services in order to deliver its economic regulatory functions such as setting efficient prices and promoting competition. Monitor and CQC will need to work closely together on some issues, but their remits are distinct; Monitor carries out economic regulation, while the CQC is responsible for assuring quality and safety. Quality and patient safety remain paramount so providers must register with the CQC according to the services they provide. Providers will have a joint licence overseen by both Monitor and CQC, to maintain essential levels of safety and quality and to ensure effective competition and the continuity of essential services.

Market stimulation and the third sector

One of the main roles of the market in health and social care is the way the third sector may be able to expand to offer some services that are valued by communities, especially but not only for minority ethnic groups. As the austerity measures have bitten during 2011 and into 2012 many voluntary and third-sector organisations have lost funding. Many of these organisations were under-funded in the first place and existed because communities wanted services and support that was acceptable and meaningful to them, perhaps for religious or cultural reasons. In Chapter 4 on public and patient involvement we saw the importance of working with groups from minority communities in a way that respects their different and diverse cultures.

During 2008–09 and subsequently the Local Government Agency (LGA) Ideas and Development Agency Office (I&DeA) of the Third Sector in the Cabinet Office developed a series of eight 'Principles' that were to be understood as providing the basis of a renewed relationship with the third sector, and should underlie any programme of work with the third sector and voluntary bodies. These form a valuable relationship between statutory and third-sector agencies and demand a renewal of that relationship. The principles were endorsed by government and are both sets of values as well as relevant to other commissioning tasks, and provide a useful guide and a check on commissioning processes.

The eight principles of good commissioning (I&DeA, 2008) describe:

1. *Understanding the needs of users and other communities by ensuring that, alongside other consultations, you engage with the third-sector organisations, as advocates, to access their specialist knowledge.* This principle ensures that third-sector organisations are always fully involved, recognising that they have knowledge that is essential to commissioning.

2. *Consulting potential provider organisations, including those from the third sector and local experts, well in advance of commissioning new services, working with them to set priority outcomes for that service.* This has been previously and may in future be contentious as it demands that the third sector (and, by extension, other organisations in the independent sector) is engaged in understanding the role of their organisation in commissioning and providing, and in developing specifications for the service to be commissioned. Private organisations may not like the way that the third sector is involved, but they have been in the vanguard of demanding values-based approach.

3. *Putting outcomes for users at the heart of the strategic planning process.* This is uncontentious although the reality is more complex. Service users should be at the *heart* of the planning process – which may be interpreted as directly and deeply involved and participating in strategic planning. If we really mean this it changes the way that commissioners make decisions!

4. *Mapping the fullest practical range of providers with a view to understanding the contribution they could make to delivering those outcomes.* Mapping *the fullest practical range* of providers requires a process for knowing who the providers are who could offer the service under discussion, contacting them, understanding their skills experience and the outcomes they offer, and seeking their interest in possibly tendering for the work. This is of course hugely work-intensive and yet is a way to ensure that (a) all those who may have a contribution can make it, (b) enables commissioners to meet competition requirements, and (c) obtains the best alternative for service users.

5. *Considering investing in the capacity of the provider base, particularly those working with hard-to-reach groups.* One of the most contested values, or imperatives, is the importance placed on capacity building the third sector especially. Private-sector providers may react to what may be perceived as favouritism or unfair practices. In practice, PCT clusters, CCGs and Health and Well-being Boards have the right to discover and develop possible sources of appropriate provider expertise.

6. *Ensuring contracting processes are transparent and fair, facilitating the involvement of the broadest range of suppliers, including considering subcontracting and consortia building, where appropriate.* Similar to the point in 4 above, this principle suggests that all tendering and contracting processes should be made available to all organisations, in ways that they can access and at reasonable times and places.

7. *Ensuring long-term contracts and risk-sharing, wherever appropriate, as ways of achieving efficiency and effectiveness.* This is particularly appropriate to the third sector as their ability to absorb risk is generally much less than independent organisations.

8. *Seeking feedback from service users, communities and providers in order to review the effectiveness of the commissioning process in meeting local needs.* This should be *de rigeur* for all commissioners and providers!

These principles were enshrined in a Compact signed by many local authorities with Councils for Voluntary Service or similar bodies. Although many PCTs do not have direct Compact agreements with the voluntary and third sector, they have been realised through Local Area Agreements and Local Strategic Partnerships. The new Compact (published in December 2010) is rather different. Five 'principles' underpin a detailed set of undertakings or commitments for the government and 'civil society organisations' (which includes charities, social enterprises, voluntary and community groups):

- a strong, diverse and independent civil society;
- effective and transparent design and development of policies, programmes and public services;
- responsive and high-quality programmes and services;
- clear arrangements for managing changes to programmes and services; and
- an equal and fair society. (Cabinet Office, 2010)

Many of the topics covered relate to the original I&DeA principles. Section 2 (effective and transparent design and development) enshrines the most important values: ensuring that social, environmental, and economic value (social value) forms a standard part of designing, developing and delivering policies, programmes and services; considering social impact; removal of barriers to action, and early notice of consultations. Section 3 includes the values of: opening up new markets to enable third sector organisations more opportunity; and ensuring well-managed and transparent application and tendering processes.

Many of these organisations have a business model that is time-limited. The pattern is one in which a programme is developed, plateaux for a short period and then declines rapidly, sometimes precipitously, when the funding ceases. The challenge will be to develop a business model that uses collated individual budgets to create a business model that is sustainable and meets the values of the participants or customers. When funding is renegotiated each year (or perhaps for a social care individual budget, every three years by social services) there will be a carefully designed programme to ensure that providers, offering components of care, are able to create a long-term sustainable approach.

Social enterprise

Social enterprises are organisations with social objectives where the main motivation is achieving a set of objectives for the community rather than the financial 'bottom line'. Any surpluses generated are reinvested to improve the business rather than being handed to shareholders in the form of dividends on investment. However, social enterprises can be both non-profit and profit-making. There is no reason in principle why an organisation should not make a surplus; it is the way the surplus is used that distinguishes social enterprises from private companies. Consequently social enterprises can be charities, companies limited by guarantee, community interest companies with an asset lock, or cooperatives.

Each of these vehicles offers slightly different advantages (and disadvantages) depending on the role it is to play. Some very large companies are social enterprises. Fairtrade, the Big Issue, Jamie Oliver's Fifteen, The Eden Project in Cornwall, or the Co-op are all social enterprises. A social enterprise is 'a business that trades to tackle social problems, improve communities, people's life chances, or the environment ... It's this combination of doing business and doing good that makes social enterprise one of the most exciting and fast-growing movements' (Social Enterprise Coalition, 2011).

Many social enterprises are small local businesses, but others have become large enough to tackle significant contracts and to challenge the private sector and other large public-sector bodies for contracts. Although there has been a great deal of encouragement from government, and useful publications (such as that from the Social Enterprise Coalition/Hempsons Solicitors, 2007), some enterprises are finding this difficult as health and social care authorities tender for care service providers. For example, a pioneering social enterprise, Central Surrey Health (CSH), is contracted to deliver community nursing and therapy services on behalf of the NHS and other organisations (e.g. Surrey County Council) to the 280,000 population of central Surrey. CSH is a not-for-profit organisation, owned by its employees, and was the first social enterprise to devolve from the NHS in 2006. Unfortunately, a recent local contract was awarded to the private sector, but it is likely CSH will continue to grow.

Social enterprises offer a way of engaging minority groups and others in tackling services for their own communities about which they know more than anyone. By working with these companies it may be possible both to engage the minority community in values-based commissioning, and to offer them the chance to provide services that they have identified (subject to appropriate rules about conflicts of interest). They will understand their community and its needs and be able to work with community members more effectively than many statutory or private providers.

Conclusion: values and the market

The market holds different values to those of public organisations. A quasi-market or social market does exist, but as we have seen it runs the risk that private organisations will cry foul, except in rare circumstances, if tenders are not let on a level playing field. Community groups hold differing values to private organisations, which increasingly will use the present laws to gain advantage. Many community groups and social enterprises are small, do not have staff able to give up time to write tenders, often hear of opportunities late, and will not cut wages and benefits to the legal minima. While it is possible for public authorities to provide resources to build capacity, and to favour those who have identified a need and a solution, it can be tricky. Any further development of the 'Big Society' needs to recognise the importance that social enterprises place on community values rather than the financial bottom line. In some places (such as Suffolk) alternative structures are emerging that enable private- and third-sector organisations to work together through subcontract relationships. Suffolk's commissioners are now known as 'market shapers', seeking to capacity build and guide the third sector while remaining true to competitive tendering requirements. Market stimulation has real opportunities for the third sector, but it must be recognised that not every organisation is fit to take part.

Chapter 11

Values-based leadership

Introduction

To be effective, values-based practice demands leadership that ensures the values of all those involved are obtained and used to decide on the right commissioning programmes. We have seen the importance of priority setting and resource allocation and we have supported the Department of Health Right Care programme that places an emphasis on programme budgeting and marginal analysis (PBMA) (Brambleby *et al.*, 2010) and mechanisms for making rational decisions about priorities. Those priorities usually address groups if not whole communities; and we were concerned that the Right Care programme did not emphasise enough the need for values to be incorporated formally and widely in the decisions taken.

Values-based leadership supports the importance of V-BP. As we shall see, there are a number of important processes that support V-BP and go beyond those correctly suggested by the Right Care team. If we are to have a values-based system, what do we need to do to ensure that it is effective? First we need to enshrine values diversity in the process of capturing values; and second, to use values diversity to provide the framework for reviewing the evidence and the background information on which to make commissioning decisions.

Commissioners will not be able to do everything, either straightaway, or possibly at all. Commissioners, especially in the dog days of the coming two years or so characterised by resource shortages multiplied by market expansion, will be hard-pressed to do many of the resource-allocation processes well. Pursuing some of them will be sufficient if that provides useful lessons on which later to base further improvements. Each CCG or PCT cluster, or indeed each Health and Well-being Board, needs to have a values proposition and a values discipline. We suggest 'values' as this is not simply about considering a 'value chain', that assists with obtaining the best *financial value* from the organisation, but is concerned with *values*. The literature on value is awash with discussions of the value chain, especially Porter's value chain analysis model (Porter, 1985), the value stream within lean thinking (Ohno, 1988), and value-mapping that considers the value-added and non-value added stages of a production line (Rother and Shock, 2003). On the other hand, a 'blue ocean' strategy (van Assen *et al.*, 2009, p. 11) will focus on what customers value, which is not solely cost.

'Blue ocean' strategies mainly assist firms to create new markets by making the competition irrelevant, capturing new demand and aligning the whole system in pursuit of differentiation and low cost (Kim and Mauborgne, 1997), but this is of interest to the health service and social care. The cost trade-offs of the coming few years will require a different way of thinking. Let us take a specific example, say a neurological long-term condition. The questions we need to ask are as follows.

- Which aspects of the present system (the care pathway, or the hospital service) can we remove, without causing a difficulty for the patient?
- Are there aspects of the care package that can be reduced – such as the frequency of visits to a clinic, or the support that is provided into the home?
- Are there aspects of the package that should be, or indeed must be, raised well above the expected standard – such as the use of tele-medicine to ensure that a patient is and remains safe at home?
- Are there additional factors that the health service has never offered? These may be available because of technological innovation, improvements in medicines, or simply ideas whose time has come!

Values space

By asking all patients and service users these questions, and by engaging the staff of the service (hospital, community and primary care, and social care providers), we will obtain a rich picture of the present service that is amenable to change. We will as a by-product either ask questions directly or reveal through analysis information on the values held by patients and service users. In thinking about these questions we must recognise that the values of the individual will be both idiosyncratic and extremely important, and may not fit within the values envelope of the group of similar service users, or the community, or indeed the population.

On the left-hand side of Figure 11.1 is the stylised ideal profile of values: the individuals values fit within that of the group, which in turn fits within those of the community, and those fit within the population perspective. Unfortunately, as we know, individuals (and groups) can be idiosyncratic. The non-idealised values map may look more like that on the right, where individual values may be squeezed into the values space allowed (taking everything into account), but does not agree with any of the communities' values. In practice this map is less about sets of values as about the numbers of those holding those values. Alternatively, therefore, we might argue that the diagram should be drawn the other way

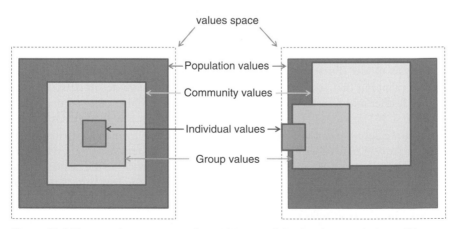

Figure 11.1 There may be many more values within a population but the agreed values will be very small (see Figure 11.2).

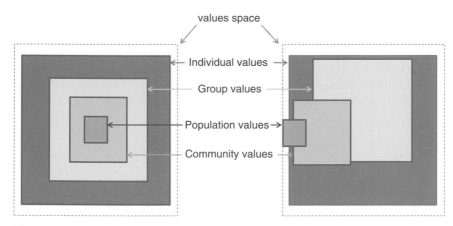

Figure 11.2 The values space shows many more individual *independent* values than in the group, community or population.

(Figure 11.2). Here we see that it is the population that has a small number of *agreed* values (by virtue of seeking acceptance from so many differing people), the community a few more, the group more again and it is the individual who has the widest set of possibly relevant values that need to be taken into account in deciding on ways of providing care.

Of course, we will need to resolve the dilemmas this poses. This will require, first, a longer discussion about the way that values are identified and understood; and second, a focus on the practical recognition of individual values in the wider scope of health and social care. From a leadership perspective, three of those core values are: operational excellence, which is of itself a further set of values; 'product' leadership, offering the best treatment or care arrangement that is available (and, in a competitive world being the first to do so!); and, customer intimacy, being dependable and responsive to customer needs (Treacy and Wiersema, 1995).

Operational excellence suggests that commissioners, just as providers, operate on 'lean' methodology, and obtain a balance between the population perspective (for efficiency) and the individual perspective (for personalisation). Being a product leader in health and social care requires an organisation to be recognised as resourceful and innovative. This may be risky. Customer 'intimacy' not only demands that commissioners know their patients and service users, and their values, but engage patients in patient- (or service user-) driven innovation. Their focus should be on exceeding patient and service user expectations, retaining patients (as customers rather than as 'patients'), achieving lifetime outcomes that are the best possible, and a reliable service (van Assen *et al.*, 2009). Choosing between the three core values may be necessary as they can be in conflict, but alternately a good commissioner will want to maximise gain from all three.

Most importantly, this changes the relationship between the health and/or social care commissioner to one that is closer, longer-term, instinctual, and not dissimilar to the relationship that FTs have or are encouraged to have with members and service users. By focusing on the long-term needs of patients and service users not only will it lead patients to a better understanding of the way that health and social care commissioning operates, but it may help to transform the relationship when it comes to serious decisions about ward or hospital closures and other significant events.

Competing values

Competing or differing values (between professional health and social care staff, patients and services users, carers, and the general public), may be reflected in the commissioning organisation (the CCG, the Health and Well-being Board, or other arrangement) to its advantage. 'Walking the talk' aligns the process and the intention. Three elements relate the effectiveness of the organisation to its process (Quinn and Rohrbaugh, 1983):

- internal compared to external focus;
- flexibility compared with stability; and
- process compared with outcome goals.

Each of these is a creative tension to be resolved. Internally, an organisation has staff and policies; externally, it has relationships with patients and service users. Ensuring that the two are in harmony is a challenge worth making explicit. The 'boundaryless organisation' is here made real (Ashenas *et al.*, 1995). All commissioners are simultaneously at the centre and at the edge of the organisation. Each GP practice, for example, will act for the best of their patients while seeking the best for all (Figure 11.3).

Flexibility and stability are often in tension: retaining control (such matters as enterprise audit, governance or probity) must be balanced with enabling autonomy and initiative in working with patients to achieve innovative solutions. Having the right arrangements will free staff to use their initiative within a 'loose – tight' framework that is at once reassuring yet provides resilient boundaries. The process – outcome distinction brings into sharp focus the tendency in complex organisations, especially ones where there are difficult decisions to make, for processes to become goals in themselves (van Assen *et al.*, 2009). This detracts from the objective of identifying values, and encourages the organisation to spend large amounts of time on identifying values at the expense of *using* those values to decide on commissioning intentions.

This model helps to understand the hidden or 'unseen' values for which 'peoples programmes, policies and organisations live and die' (van Assen *et al.*, 2009) and demonstrates the process by which the organisations' values can be made explicit and disaggregated in order to inform negotiation with the values of patients, service users and the public. Some of those values can be identified through focus groups, workshops and seminars, properly facilitated. But only by becoming a learning organisation can the values of the organisation

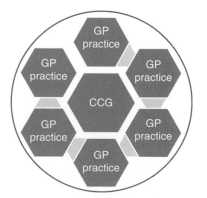

Figure 11.3 Each GP practice in a CCG is at the edge of the CCG as well as entirely part of it.

be translated into a values programme that is then checked against the values of the patients and service users in a way that changes the commissioning strategy. A learning organisation requires a number of factors: systems thinking; personal strength; mental models; a shared vision; and team learning (Senge, 1990). These all impact on the ideas and processes described in the previous paragraphs and enable us to see how the programme we discussed above is made unambiguous.

Systems thinking

Systems thinking concerns holistic perspectives and interconnectedness – the point we have discussed previously (in Chapter 9 especially). As we saw, one of the important aspects of systems thinking is in providing opportunities for modelling which then enable a range of options to be developed and tested without the expense of doing it 'for real'. Models can sometimes bring out the complexity of what may be thought at first a relatively simple system. Whole systems are essential to the task of creating a fundamentally economic and effective health and social care programme, and demonstrate in practice that there is no more effective or economic arrangement of resources than an integrative provider structure. Unnecessary boundaries between providers are expensive, although some are needed.

However, there is more to systems thinking than Senge offers. Senge's approach to the learning organisation lacks the quality of 'ethical alertness' (Flood, 1999, p. 61). Ethical alertness comes from thinking systemically; and efficiency and effectiveness from considering the total system (Churchman, 1971 in Flood, 1999, p. 63). However, more importantly for Churchman, the principles of systemic thinking relate to our concern for values and values-based practice. The principles state that the systems approach:

- begins when you first see the world through the eyes of another;

- goes on the discover that every world view is terribly restricted;

- contains no experts; and

- is not a bad idea!

Churchman's systemic thinking is thus 'deeply moral', and reflects values-based practice; he was 'relentless in his quest for critically reflective and moral practice' (Flood, 1999, p. 61). 'Beginning when you see the world through the eyes of another' sums up the core of values-based practice. By understanding how others see the world, we can see it better. Values-based practice incorporates the humanely purposeful approach that Churchman brought to his work and his desire to ensure that people can justify their choices and actions (Flood, 1999, p. 66). This can also be seen in the proposition of Argyris and Schon (1978) for what they call their 'theory-in-use'. To be effective, any manager needs to be open to alternatives and take action after free and informed choice of all those who have a contribution to make.

Promoting personal mastery, through personal strength or responsibility, reflects the way that organisations learn through their staff. If individuals are motivated to learn, then the organisation learns too. However, without a 'glue' or systems approach it will not achieve the breakthrough, the tipping point that ensures the organisation learns; in our case, that learning is about the values of each other and of patients and service users, other staff of the commissioner and provider organisations, and the general public. Adopting V-BP enables organisations to work through their values, develop consensus and dissensus, and use the outcome to ensure as consistent an approach with agreed derogation based on mutual trust and understanding.

Mental models are an essential feature of Senge's model of the learning organisation (Senge, 1990). By mental models, Senge suggests that these are 'deeply ingrained assumptions, generalisations, or even pictures and images that influence how we understand the world'; in other words, values. Values-based practice helps to make explicit their values by the process of building a learning organisation, in which people make expose their own values and ideals to wider scrutiny. V-BP has a crucial role in values-based commissioning, not only because it offers the opportunity to negotiate and secure the active engagement of stakeholders, but because it helps the organisation to develop its own shared values.

The final two components of Senge's outline are 'building a shared vision' and 'team learning'. The first is that leaders need to articulate a vision that will motivate staff to engage actively with the process of values identification and use; the second is that teams can learn together profitably. 'No-one is perfect but a team can be' was a refrain from 30 years ago, and is applicable today as it was then. We all have our strengths and weaknesses; we are all better at some things than others. Some learn through doing, others from books, or the internet; some are good with people, some want to work in a backroom where they can labour undisturbed. But together, teams can build on each other's strengths through mutual respect and recognition of difference (Senge, 1999).

Leadership in health and social care

Leadership is something that all can practice, but it is essential that those charged with leading a CCG or Health and Well-being Board do so in a way that provides direction and resolution. Leadership in commissioning involves a 'visible, credible, coherent and inclusive approach underpinned by a vision that all ... can share'. Leaders 'steer and influence the priorities of the local area' to achieve a coherent and agreed set of values and priorities that is accepted by all those involved (Commissioning Support Programme, 2010, p. 19).

Leadership in health and social care is vital at any time, but during the changes of the next two or three years will need to be vigorous, especially to recognise the importance of values and to reflect and refract evidence through those values. That will require an understanding of values-based practice, an acceptance that health well-being and social care is a 'frustrated continuum' (that is, at once extensive and integrated, and has discontinuities that demand attention); and a recognition of values pluralism, not just between communities of differing ethnicity, or age, or disability, but also between acute health providers, community services, social care, and the third sector. A lack of leadership and a lack of strategic coordination may be due to senior managers unable to engage adequately because of the extent of the transformation, or a lack of good information and evaluation about what is happening, or difficulties in specifying roles and relationships until the government has some clarity about the final shape of legislation and its implementation.

Leadership, and followership, will be vital. Unless CCGs have a form of distributed leadership it is possible that those practices which are not part of the leadership team will not cooperate with tough decisions, for example, to deny patients treatments of dubious worth. Leadership of Health and Well-being Boards will be critical. There is a suggestion that having fewer larger CCGs coterminus with Health and Well-being Boards will be more productive. Nonetheless, it is possible that not all councillors will agree the shape of commissioning intentions despite their stated aim of cooperation between health and social care. Where a councillor has been elected on a particular political 'platform' it will be difficult to prise him or her away from it. Consequently relationships matter in health and social care.

Minimising the number of critical relationships may help, but the complexity of the system means that political and professional values will come increasingly into contention. Only by a concerted effort to identify the values and to negotiate on those that compete will it be possible to agree an acceptable compromise way forward.

Changing the paradigm: innovation and transformation

An alternative conception of values-based commissioning recognises the importance of process innovation that leads to service user-driven innovation. For example, customer-driven innovation has become a major selling feature in USA car sales (Ulwick, 2002). Customers are encouraged to suggest ideas, changes to the specification or style of components, or innovative design cues. Not only does this glue customers to the product, but it ensures that the product includes measures, designs and components that customers want and like.

As information sharing increases, the system goes from one of technology innovation through process innovation to innovation in provision of service-user choices and user innovation. Users will often have ideas that may be helpful. This can be true especially in long-term and chronic care (mental health or neurological disorders), but increasingly we see this in other aspects of acute medicine on the one hand and social care on the other.

Figure 11.4, based on thinking radically from the American military (Adams, 2000), describes the importance of harnessed innovation to assist all those at the 'sharp end' – in the military, soldiers, but in our case, patients, service users, doctors nurses and social care staff. Choice is critical; choice made by the service user at the moment of need. That can only occur if the system is set up not just to offer choice, but to have choices available all the time, even though this may increase redundancy several-fold. For the military it is essential to have the choice of weapons at the moment of greatest need – under fire in a tight corner. Having choices available is costly and will require a careful assessment of the balance of need and provision to decide the levels of care available. Nonetheless, responsible staff working with

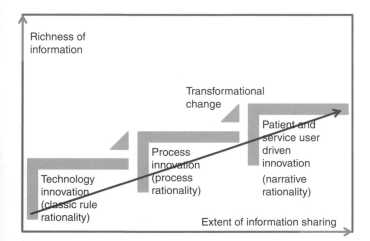

Figure 11.4 Information richness and the extent of information sharing will increase the chance of transformational innovation.

responsible service users can ensure that this is managed and reduced to the desirable minimum. The important point is the significance of process innovation. Developments of provision demand an agreed concrete but flexible process that taps into the service user values and articulates the service user view effectively. The greater the information sharing with patients and service users the greater the innovation, and likely cost savings that will result.

'Value' and 'values'

In any discussion of 'values' the notion of 'value' arises. 'Value' is a composite term that reflects the utility of the service provided in addressing health and social care need. 'Value' is used as a generic management term to describe the worth to the 'firm' or organisation, but rarely (although there are exceptions in the literature) to the customer of the 'product'. The product may be a new hip, or a nursing home placement. So what is 'value'? Is it a composite of evidence used in the real product creation, together with values made explicit? And what is a 'value-chain'?

Porter's value-chain analysis (Porter, 1985) suggests that (a) there are many factors to consider, (b) the value-chain is predicated mainly on making a profit (or surplus), and (c) is concerned with ensuring that necessary equipment, instruments and prostheses are available. 'Value in any field must be defined around the customer, not the supplier. Value must also be measured by outputs, not inputs. Hence it is patient health results that matter, not the volume of services delivered. But results are achieved at some cost. Therefore, the proper objective is ... the patient health outcomes relative to the total cost (inputs). Efficiency, then, is subsumed in the concept of value' (Porter, 2011). Much of this does not directly challenge a patient's values unless and until there is a problem with the supply chain. This may occur for a number of reasons, some of which if they happen rarely can be forgiven, but if they happen frequently will not accord with values of timeliness, relevance and appropriateness.

The value chain is thus an important factor in health care especially. In social care, 'value' is achieved in part through systems that promote 'best value', such as competitive tendering of social care provision, and in part through recognising the aspirations and life objectives of clients or service users. In mental health care 'recovery' has become the main objective. Recovery is a values-driven outcome. A patient's medium-term objectives and life goals should be the aim of the service: to provide care support and treatment that promotes those goals and meets the aspirations of the service user. In services to older people with physical disabilities the value of the service to the older person will be some variable amalgam of good quality social support with effective care for the implications of disability. The value will be a summation of the utility that is gained from the different components of care. The NHS Right Care programme believes value can be increased in two ways.

- 'By doing things better and cheaper – quality improvement improves outcome; productivity improvement reduces resource usage;
- By doing the right things – that is, shifting spend from lower value interventions to higher value interventions and ensuring that patients receive appropriate interventions.' (QIPP Right Care, 2011)

These different components can be identified and a value applied. It will be seen that the summation will be the personally appropriate list of 'values' with a method of quantification that allows them to be collated. Some will not be comparable and thus will not be amenable to collation by reasonable means. However, others can be given a value and summed to generate either a comparative value (e.g. of one patient or service user to another) or to show the value outcome for contractual purposes. In this way the 'value' of an individual budget can be at least compared even if the absolute value is not readily available. This then allows value for money calculations to be made, assuming that we know the cost of the contract either for individuals or groups. Amartya Sen suggests that the plurality of interpretation of individual preferences is indeed a strength. 'In different types of evaluative arguments about . . . social decisions' he suggests, 'the richness of the variety of interpretations permits the theory to invoke different features of the individual, depending on the context' (Sen, 2002, p. 304).

Engaging with values and preferences in social choices can be a little more relaxed than engaging with the evidence, even though much of the evidence has a values base. Although 'individual values can and do change in the process of decision making' (Buchanan, 1954, p. 120 quoted in Sen, 2002, p. 454), there is much to commend plurality and recognise that individuals have a wide variety of values, beliefs and preferences; it is unnecessary to demand a coherent value-set in order to achieve values-based practice.

Conclusion

Leadership in health and social care demands a values-based perspective. By engaging patients and service users to drive innovation we get two things: new ideas that change the way professional staff view the world; and committed and motivated customers who feel involved and listened to. The management literature has a lot to say to us about how we can do things better. However, fundamentally, working with patients and service users effectively (closely, supportively, honestly) will achieve more than making decisions about health and social care with no input from the people for whom the service was established. A genuine attempt to work with customers will pay dividends many times over.

Endnote

Values-based commissioning (V-BC) is a necessary complement to evidence-based practice (E-BP). By bringing the two together we obtain both the values of those who plan, provide and use services, with the evidence, both good and bad, about what does or does not work. Thus V-BC will demand that the evidence is filtered through a V-BC mesh of relevant values; and this ensures that patients and service users accept more readily what the evidence tells us.

We have seen in the book the challenge of establishing V-BC, especially at a time of austerity. Some will conclude that it is too expensive in time or resources. Others may feel it is valuable but only when we have time; at the moment, it is a luxury that we cannot afford. To these sceptics we say: V-BC will help enormously in ensuring that patients and service users accept the restrictions on services as long as they have been fully involved in making those decisions and the decisions are genuinely based on an analysis of competing values. This will be true for those services which are deemed too expensive or for which there is insufficient positive evidence; but conversely where there is not good evidence, V-BC allows commissioners to buy innovative treatments that accord with patients and service users values.

This book should be read in conjunction with Fulford *et al.* (2012, forthcoming), in the same CUP series, on the principles and practice of values-based commissioning. Cross-referring their rigorous and comprehensive approach to the detail of values-based practice will enable the approach adopted here to be put into practice locally.

The discussion has taken an overview of V-BC in a range of disciplines: in health and social care management generally, in health economics, in rationality and systems, in public health, integrative care, priority setting, outcomes, market stimulation and leadership. Each discussion is linked to each of the others. Each chapter builds the case for values-based practice. The consideration of the reforms in England will almost certainly be out of date before the book is printed, but the discussion focuses on important issues of principle that will continue to excite interest. Not everything on each topic is concerned with values; but there is sufficient evidence about the importance of values-thinking in each chapter to create an unstoppable momentum for values-based practice to be given a much greater presence in health and social care practice.

References

NHS Constitution – Interactive version. http://www.nhs.uk/choiceintheNHS/Rightsandpledges/NHSConstitution/Documents/nhs-constitution-interactive-version-march-2010.pdf. 2010.

Guiding Principles for EU legislation. Department of Business, Innovation and Skills. 2011.

Localism goes to the Lords. http://www.curtinandco.com/news/full/The-Localism-Bill-goes-to-the-Lords. 2011.

Picture of values. http://mommyblues.wordpress.com/2009/12/30/identify-your-top-5-values-and-watch-your-true-self-emerge/. 2011

Supporting evidence-based, best value healthcare decisions – Clinical commissioning groups: commissioning for the future. http://www.sph.nhs.uk/what-we-do/supporting-evidence-based-best-value-healthcare-decisions. 2011.

The Equalities Act 2010. Home Office.

Herfindahl Index. http://en.wikipedia.org/wiki/Herfindahl_index, accessed 30 June 2011.

Health expectancy: Living longer in poor health. Office of National Statistics. 2011.

Cornell University Policy on Equalities. 2011.

Abma, T. A., Nierse, C. and Widdershoven, G. A. M. 2009. Patients as partners in responsive research: Methodological notions for collaborations in mixed research teams. *Qualitative Health Research*, **19**, 401.

Adams T. K. 2000. *The Real Military Revolution*. Parameters **30**[3], US Army War College, 1–13.

Agich G. J. 1993. *Autonomy and Long-Term Care*. New York, Oxford University Press.

Airoldi M. and Morton A. 2009. Adjusting life for health or disability: stylistic differences or substantial issue? *Health Economics*, **18**(11), 1237–1247

Airoldi M., *et al.* Presentation to ESRC seminar, 2009. Unpublished.

Anchor and 29 others. Think Local, Act Personal: Next Steps for Transforming Adult Social Care. 2011. London, Think Local Act Personal.

Appleby J., Crawford R. and Emmerson C. 2009. *How Cold Will it Be? Prospects for NHS Funding: 2011–17*. London: Kings Fund & Institute for Fiscal Studies.

Appleby J., Raleigh V., Frosini F., Bevan G., Gao H. and Lyscom T. 2011. *Variations in Health Care: The Good, the Bad and the Inexplicable*. London: Kings Fund.

Argyris C. and Schon D. 1978. *Organizational Learning: A Theory of Action Perspective*. Reading, MA: Addison-Wesley.

Aristotle. 2000. *Nicomachean Ethics*. Cambridge: Cambridge University Press.

Arnesen T. and Nord E. 1999. The value of DALY life: Problems with ethics and validity of disability adjusted life years. *British Medical Journal* **319**, 1423–1425.

Arrow K. J. 1984. *Social Choice and Justice*. Oxford, Blackwell.

Ashenas R., Ulrich D., Jich T. and Herr S. 1995. *The Boundaryless Organization: Breaking the Chains of Organizational Structure*. San Francisco, CA: Jossey-Bass.

Association of Public Health Observatories. 2011. *APHO Small Area Indicators for Joint Strategic Needs Assessment*. Available at: http://www.apho.org.uk/RESOURCE/VIEW.ASPX?RID=87735

BBC. 2011. 'Four arrests after patient abuse caught on film'. Available at: www.bbc.co.uk/news/uk-13548222, accessed 31 May 2011.

Beauchamp T. L. and Childress J. F. 2001. *Principles of Biomedical Ethics*. Oxford, Oxford University Press.

Bero L. A., Grilli R., Grimshaw J. M., *et al.* 1998. Getting research findings into practice. Closing the gap between research and practice: an overview of systematic reviews of interventions to promote the implementation of research findings. *British Medical Journal* **317**, 465.

Birrell F. N., Hassell A. B., Jones P. W. and Dawes P. T. 2011. How does the Short Form 36 Health Questionnaire (SF-36) in Rheumatoid Arthritis (RA) relate to RA outcome measures and SF-36 population values? A cross-sectional study. *Clinical Rheumatology* **19**(3), 195–199.

Blackstone, Sir William. 1753. *Commentaries on the Laws of England in Four Books, vol. 1* [1753]. Edition used: *Commentaries on the Laws of England in Four Books. Notes selected from the editions of Archibold, Christian, Coleridge, Chitty, Stewart, Kerr, and others, Barron Field's Analysis, and Additional Notes, and a Life of the Author by George Sharswood.* In 2 volumes. (Philadelphia: J.B. Lippincott Co., 1893). Vol. 1, Books I and II.

Bradshaw J. 1972. A taxonomy of social need. *New Society*, 640–643.

Brambleby P., Jackson A. and Stewart I. 2010, *The Third Annual Population Review: Commissioning for Health Improvement Using programme budgeting and marginal analysis to deliver quality, innovation productivity and prevention.* London: NHS/Department of Health.

Brown H. 1990. *Rationality*. London: Routledge.

Brown M. M, Brown G. C. and Sharma S. 2005. *Evidence-Based to Value-Based Medicine.* Chicago, IL: American Medical Association Press.

Buchanan J. M. 1954. Social choice, democracy and free markets. *Journal of Political Economy* **62**, 114–123.

Bursztajn H. J., Feinbloom R. I., Hamm R. M. and Brodsky A. 1990. *Medical Choices, Medical Chances: How Patients, Families and Physicians Can Cope with Uncertainty.* New York/London: Routledge.

Cabinet Office. 2010. *The Compact: The Coalition Government and civil society organisations working effectively in partnership for the benefit of communities and citizens in England.* London: Author.

Care Quality Commission. 2011. *Count me in Census 2010.* London: Care Quality Commission.

Carson D., Clay H. and Stern R. 2010. Primary Care and Emergency Departments: Report from the Primary Care Foundation. Available at: www.dh.gov.uk/en/Publicationsandstatistics/Publications/PublicationsPolicyAndGuidance/DH_113694.

Centre for the Evaluative Clinical Sciences. 2005. *Dartmouth Atlas (2005). 'Cardiac Surgery'.* Dartmouth, NH: Dartmouth Atlas of Health Care.

Chang R. 1997. *Incommensurability, Incomparability, and Practical Reason.* Boston, MA: Harvard College.

Cherrett K. 2010. *Total Place: A Tantalising Truth.* London: Guardian Public Leaders Network.

Churchman C. W. 1971. *The Design of Inquiring Systems: Basic Concepts of Systems and Organisations.* New York, NY: Basic Books.

Clark, H., Gough, H. and Macfarlane, A. 2004. *Making Direct Payments Work for Older People.* York: Joseph Rowntree Foundation.

Commissioning Support Programme. 2010. *Good Commissioning: Principles and Practice.* London: Commissioning Support Programme.

Conway M. 2007. The value of values – do they go deep enough? *In: Medicine of the Person: Faith, Science and Values in Health Care Provision,* Cox J, Campbell A V, and Fulford K W M, eds. London: Jessica Kingsley, pp. 70–80.

Cooperation and Competition Panel. 2011. *Review of the Operation of 'Any Willing Provider' for the Provision of Routine Elective Care. Final Report.* London: CCP.

Coulter A. and Collins A. 2011. *Making Shared Decision-Making a Reality. No Decision About Me, Without Me.* www.kingsfund.org.uk/publications. London: The Kings Fund and the Foundation for Informed Medical Decision Making.

Coulter, A. 2006. Can patients assess the quality of health care? *British Medical Journal* **333**(7557), 1–2.

Cronje R. and Fullan A. 2003. Evidence-based medicine: toward a new definition of 'rational' medicine. *Health: An Interdisciplinary Journal for the Social Study of Health, Illness and Medicine* **7**(3), 353–369.

Curry N., Goodwin N., Naylor C. and Robertson R. 2010. *Practice-based Commissioning: Reinvigorate, Replace or Abandon?* London: Kings Fund.

Curry R. 2011. Locke and the Declaration of Independence. www.thomasbrewton.com/index.php/weblog/why_happiness, accessed 1 April 2012.

Curry R. 2011. Locke and the Declaration of Independence.. www.kingsfund.org.uk/publications. London: The Kings Fund and the Foundation for Informed Medical Decision Making.

Curtis J. R., Patrick D. L., Shannon S. E., *et al.* 2001. The family conference as a focus to improve communication about end-of-life care in the intensive care unit: opportunities for improvement. *Critical Care Medicine* **29**(2), 26–33.

Daniels N. 2000. Accountability for reasonableness. *British Medical Journal* **321**, 1300–1301.

Daniels N. and Sabin J. E. 1997. Limits to health care: fair procedures, democratic deliberation and the legitimacy problems of insurers. *Philosophy and Public Affairs*, **26**, 303–350.

Daniels N. and Sabin J. 2002. *Setting Limits Fairly: Can We Learn to Share Medical Resources?* Oxford/New York: Oxford University Press.

Daykin N., Evans D., Petsoulas C. and Sayers A. 2007. Evaluating the impact of patient and public involvement initiatives on UK health services: a systematic review. *Evidence and Policy* **3**(1), 47–65.

de Wit M. P. T., Berlo S. E., Aanerud G. J., *et al.* 2011. Recommendation: European League Against Rheumatism recommendations for the inclusion of patient representatives in scientific projects. *Annals of the Rheumatic Diseases* **70**: 722–726.

Delap C. 1998. *Making Better Decisions. Report of an IPPR symposium on citizens' juries and other methods of public involvement.* London: IPPR.

Department of Communities and Local Government. 2008. *Creating Strong, Safe and Prosperous Communities: Statutory Guidance.* London: DCLG. Available at: http://www.communities.gov.uk/publications/localgovernment/strongsafeprosperous

Department of Communities and Local Government. 2011. Proposals to introduce a Community Right to Challenge: Consultation paper. Available at: http://www.communities.gov.uk/documents/localgovernment/pdf/1835810.pdf. London: DCLG.

Department of Health. 2005. *Delivering Race Equality in Mental Health Care: An Action Plan for Reform Inside and Outside Services and the Government's Response to the Independent Inquiry into the Death of David Bennett.* London: Department of Health.

Department of Health. 2007. *Commissioning Framework.* London: Department of Health.

Department of Health. 2009. *New Horizons: A Shared Vision for Mental Health.* London: Department of Health.

Department of Health. 2010a. *Equity and Excellence: Liberating the NHS.* London: Department of Health.

Department of Health. 2010b. *A Vision for Adult Social Care: Capable Communities and Active Citizens.* London: Author.

Department of Health. 2011a. *Transparency in Outcomes – A Framework for the NHS.* London: Department of Health.

Department of Health. 2011b. *Transparency in Outcomes: A Framework for Adult Social Care: A Consultation on Proposals.* London: Department of Health.

Department of Health. 2011c. *The NHS Outcomes Framework 2011/12.* London: Department of Health.

Department of Health. 2011d. *Healthy Lives, Healthy People: Update and Way Forward.* London: Department of Health.

DIY Citizens Jury. 2003a. *Jury Verdizt.* Newcastle upon Tyre: DIY Jury Steering Group and the Polizy Ethics and Life Sciences Research Institute, University of Newcastle.

Dolan P., Cookson R. and Ferguson B. 1999. Effect of discussion and deliberation on the public's views of priority setting in health care: focus group study. *British Medical Journal* **318**, 916.

Donabedian A. 1988. The quality of care – how can it be assessed? *Journal of the American Medical Association* **260**: 1743–1748.

Dowling B. 2000. *GPs and Purchasing in the NHS: The Internal Market and Beyond.* Aldershot: Ashgate.

Drake R. E., Goldman H. H., Leff H. S., *et al.* 2001. Implementing evidence-based practices in routine mental health service settings. *Psychiatric Services* **52**(2): 179–182.

Drummond M. F., Stoddart G. L. and Torrance G. W. 1987. *Methods for the Economic Evaluation of Health Care Programmes*. Oxford: Oxford University Press.

Eagger S., Desser A. and Brown C. 2005. Learning values in healthcare? *Journal of Holistic Healthcare*, **2**(3), 25–30.

Einsiedel E. F. and Eastlick D. L. 2000. Consensus conferences as deliberative democracy: a communications perspective. *Science Communication* **21**(4), 323–343.

Ernst and Young and Frontier Economics. 2011. *Understanding Health Care Markets: A PCT Guide to Market Analysis and Market Management*. London.

Flood R. L. 1999. *Rethinking the Fifth Discipline*. London: Routledge.

Forder J., Netten A., Caiels J., Smith J. and Malley J. 2007. *Measuring Outcomes in Social Care: Conceptual Development and Empirical Design*. Canterbury: University of Kent/LSE/University of Manchester, PSSRU.

Foresight, The. Govt. Office for Science. 2009. *Mental Capital and Well-being Final Project Report*. London: The Government Office for Science.

Fraenkel L., Bogardus S. T., Concato J., Felson D. T. and Wittink D. R. 2004. Patient preferences for treatment of rheumatoid arthritis. *Annals of the Rheumatic Diseases* **63**, 1372–1378.

Franklin J. 1998. *Social Policy and Social Justice: The IPPR Reader*. Oxford: Polity Press with Blackwell.

Fraser N. and Honneth A. 2003. *Redistribution and Recognition*. London: Verso.

Friedli L. 2009. *Mental Health, Resilience and Inequalities*. Copenhagen: World Health Organisation.

Fulford, K. W. M. 1989. *Moral Theory and Medical Practice*. Cambridge: Cambridge University Press.

Fulford K. W. M. 2004. Ten principles of values-based medicine. In: *The Philosophy of Psychiatry: A Companion*, Radden J, ed. New York, NY: Oxford University Press, pp. 205–234.

Fulford K. W. M. 2011a. *Moral Theory and Medical Practice*. Cambridge: Cambridge University Press.

Fulford K. W. M. 2011b. Dissent and dissensus: the limits of consensus in psychiatry. In: *Consensus Formation in Health Care Ethics*, ten Have H A M J and Saas H-M, eds. Amsterdam: Kluwer, pp. 175–192.

Fulford K. W. M., Dickenson D. and Murray, T. H. 2002. *Healthcare Ethics and Human Values: An Introductory Text with Readings and Case Studies*. Oxford: Blackwell.

Fulford K. W. M., Peile E., & Carroll H. forthcoming 2012. *Essential Values-based Practice: Clinical Stories linking Science with People*. Cambridge: Cambridge University Press.

Goetghebeur M. M., Wagner M., Khoury H., Levitt R. J., Erickson L. J. and Rindress D. 2008. Evidence and value: impact on DEcisionMaking – the EVIDEM framework and potential applications. *BMC Health Services Research* **8**(270).

Gooberman-Hill R. and Calnan M. 2008. Citizens' juries in planning research priorities: process, engagement and outcome. *Health Expectations* **11**(3), 272–281.

Goodacre L. J. and Goodacre J. A. 2004. Factors influencing the beliefs of patients with rheumatoid arthritis regarding disease-modifying medication. *Rheumatology* **43**(5), 583–586.

Greenhalgh T. 1999. Narrative-based medicine in an evidence-based world. *British Medical Journal*, **318** (7179), 323 ff.

Habermas J. 1984. *The Theory of Communicative Action: Reason and the Rationalization of Society, Vol. 1*. Boston, MA: Beacon Press.

Ham C. and Pickard S. 2011. *Tragic Choices in Health Care: The Case of Child B*. London: Kings Fund Publishing.

Hare R. M. 1952. *The Language of Morals*. Oxford: Oxford University Press.

Harris J. 1987. QALYfying the value of life. *Journal of Medical Ethics*, **13**(3), 117–123.

Harris J. 1995. Double jeopardy and the veil of ignorance – a reply. *Journal of Medical Ethics*, **21**, 151–157.

Haynes R., Devereaux P. and Guyatt G. 2002. Physicians' and patients' choices in evidence based practice. *British Medical Journal* **324**, 1350.

Heginbotham C., Ham C., Cochrane M. and Richards J. 1992. *Purchasing Dilemmas*. London: Kings Fund.

Hewletta S., Smith A. P. and Kirwana J. R. 2001. Extended report: Values for function in rheumatoid arthritis: Patients, professionals, and public. *Annals of the Rheumatic Diseases* **60**, 928–933.

Hippisley-Cox J. 2009. *Health Inequalities in Primary Care: Effect of Spearhead Primary Care Trusts 2002–2009*. Nottingham: Department of Health.

Hirschman A. O. 1964. The paternity of an index. *The American Economic Review (American Economic Association)*, 54(5), 761.

Hirshfield J. 2008. *Hiddenness, Uncertainty, Surprise: Three Generative Energies of Poetry*. Newcastle upon Tyne/Tarset, Newcastle University/Bloodaxe.

Hoffmann C., Stoyaka B. A., Nixon J., *et al.* 2002. Do health-care decision makers find economic evaluations useful? The findings of focus group Research in UK Health Authorities. *Value in Health* 5(2), 71–78.

Honigsbaum F. 1993. *Who Shall Live? Who Shall Die?* London: Kings Fund.

Honigsbaum F., Calltorp J., Ham C. and Holmstrom S. 1995. *Priority Setting Processes for Healthcare*. Abingdon, Oxford: Radcliffe Medical Press.

Hope T., Savalescu J. and Hendrick J. 2003. *Medical Ethics and the Law: The Core Curriculum*. Edinburgh: Churchill Livingston.

http: and www.ncl.ac.uk/peals/dialogues/juries.htm. 2010. *Community Jury Project*.

Hume D. 2000. *A Treatise of Human Nature*, Norton D. F. and Norton M. .J, eds, with Editor's Introduction by D. F. Norton. Oxford: Oxford University Press.

I&DeA. 2008. *Eight Principles of Good Commissioning*. London, I&DeA/Cabinet Office.

In Control. 2009, revised 2011. *Citizenship in Health: Theory to Practice*. Wythall, West Midlands: In Control.

Isaacs J. D. and Ferraccioli G. 2010. The need for personalised medicine for rheumatoid arthritis. *Annals of the Rheumatic Diseases*, 70, 4–7.

Jenkinson C., Coulter A. and Bruster S. 2002. The Picker Patient Experience Questionnaire: development and validation using data from in-patient surveys in five countries. *International Journal for Quality in Health Care* 14(5), 353–358.

Jensen U. J. and Mooney G. 1990. *Changing Values in Medical and Health Care Decision Making*. Chichester: Wiley.

Kay A. 2002. The abolition of the GP fundholding scheme: a lesson in evidence-based policy making. *British Journal of General Practice* 52, 141–144.

Keeley D. 1997. General practice fundholding and health care costs. *British Medical Journal* 315(7101), 139.

Keyes C. L. M. 2002. The mental health continuum: from languishing to flourishing in life. *Journal of Health and Behavior Research* 43, 207–222.

Kim W. C. and Mauborgne R. 1997. Value innovation – the strategic logic of high growth. *Harvard Business Review* 75, January–February, 103–112. (Collected in a book as Kim, C. 2005. *Blue Ocean Strategy*. Boston, MA: Harvard Business School Press.)

Kim-Cohen, J., Caspi, A., Moffitt, T. E., *et al.* 2003. Prior juvenile diagnoses in adults with mental disorder. *Archives of General Psychiatry* 60, 709–717.

Kings Fund. 2010. *Clinical Commissioning: What Can We Learn from Previous Commissioning Models?* Available at: http://www.kingsfund.org.uk/current_projects/the_nhs_white_paper/gp_commissioning.html.

Kitzinger J. 1995. Introducing focus groups. *British Medical Journal* 311(7000), 299–302.

Knapp M., Bauer A., Perkins M. and Snell T. 2010. *Building Community Capacity: Making an Economic Case*. London/Cambridge: PSSRU.

Last J. M. 2006. *A Dictionary of Public Health*. New York, NY: Oxford University Press.

Lawrence, V., Murray, J., Samsi, K. and Banerjee, S. 2008. Attitudes and support needs of Black Caribbean, south Asian and White British carers of people with dementia in the UK. *British Journal of Psychiatry* 193(3), 240–246.

Le Grand J., Mays N. and Mulligan J-A. 1998. *Learning from the NHS Internal Market: A Review of the Evidence*. London: Kings Fund.

Leadbeater C. 2004. *Personalisation through Participation: A New Script for Public Services*. London: Demos.

Leutz W. 1999. Five laws for integrating acute and long-term care. *Milbank Quarterly* 77(1), 77–110.

Leutz W. 2005. Reflections on integrating medical and social care: five laws revisited. *Journal of Integrated Care* **13**(5), 3–12.

Light D. W. 2011. *Effective Commissioning: Lessons from Purchasing in American Managed Care.* London: Office of Health Economics.

Lindenmeyer A., Griffiths F. and Hodson J. 2011. 'The family is part of the treatment really': a qualitative exploration of collective health narratives in families. *Health* **15**(4), 401–415.

Little M., Jordens C. F. C., Paul K., Sayers E. and Sriskandarajah D. 1999. Approval and disapproval in the narratives of colorectal cancer patients and their carers. *Health* **3**(4), 451–467.

Lockwood M. 1988, Quality of life and resource allocation. In: *Philosophy and Medical Welfare*, Bell J M and Mendus S, eds. Cambridge: Cambridge University Press.

Madsen K. M., Hvid A., Vestergaard M., *et al.* 2002. A population-based study of measles, mumps and rubella vaccination and autism. *New England Journal of Medicine* **347**(7), 1477.

Marmot M. 2010. *The Marmot Review (2010) Fair Society, Healthy Lives.* London: University College London.

Mays N. 2001. *The Purchasing of Health Care by Primary Care Organizations: An Evaluation and Guide to Future Policy.* Buckingham: Open University Press in association with the King's Fund.

McGreevy D. 2005. Risks and benefits of the single versus the triple MMR vaccine: how can health professionals reassure parents? *Perspectives in Public Health* **125**(2), 84–86.

McKibben, B. (2010) *eaarth.* New York, NY: Times Books.

Mitton C. and Donaldson C. 2004. *Priority Setting Toolkit: A Guide to the Use of Economics in Healthcare Decision Making.* London: BMJ Publications.

Mooney G. and McGuire A, eds. 1988. Economics and medical ethics in health care: an economic viewpoint. In: *Medical Ethics and Economics in Health Care.* Oxford: Oxford University Press, pp. 5–22.

Moore G. E. 2000. *Principia Ethica.* Cambridge: Cambridge University Press.

Mullen P. and Spurgeon P. 2000. *Priority Setting and the Public.* Abingdon, Oxford: Radcliffe Medical Press.

National Audit Office. 2010. *Tackling Inequalities in Life Expectancy in Areas with the Worst Health and Deprivation.* London: Department of Health and NAO.

Newbigging K. and Heginbotham C. J. 2010. *Commissioning Mental Well-being for All.* Preston: University of Central Lancashire.

NHS Confederation. 2011. Personal health budgets: the views of service users and carers. (11/8/2011).

NICE. 2008. *Community Engagement to Improve Health. Public Health Guidance 9.* London: Author.

NICE and SCIE. 2006. *Dementia: Supporting People with Dementia and their Carers in Health and Social Care.* London: NICE and SCIE.

Nord E. 1999. *Cost Value Analysis in Health Care: Making Sense of QALYs.* Cambridge: Cambridge University Press.

Office for National Statistics. 2010. *Measuring Outcomes for Public Service Users (MOPSU) Project: Outcomes of Adult Social Care Services.* London: Office of National Statistics.

Ohno, T. 1988. *The Toyota Production System: Beyond Large-scale Production.* London: Productivity Press.

Oregon Health Services Commission. 1991. *Prioritisation of Health Services.* Portland, OR: Oregon Health Services Commission.

Orr, A. H. 2011. The science of right and wrong. A review in the *New York Review of Books* 12 May 2011 of Harris, S. 2010. *The Moral Landscape: How Science Can Determine Human Values.* New York, NY: Free Press.

Pellegrino, E. D. 2005. Futility in medical decisions: the word and the concept. *HEC Forum* **17**(4), 308–318.

Pellegrino, E. D. and Thomasma, D. C. 1988. *For the Patient's Good: The Restoration of Beneficence in Health Care.* New York, NY: Oxford University Press.

Pettiti D. B. 2011. *Meta-Analysis, Decision Analysis, and Cost Effectiveness Analysis: Methods for Quantitative Synthesis in Medicine*, second edition. New York, NY: Oxford University Press.

Pickin, C., Popay, J., Staely, K., *et al.* 2002. Developing a model to enhance the capacity of statutory organisations to engage with lay communities. *Journal of Health Services Research and Policy* 7(1).

Pines A. and Aronson E. 2011. *Career Burnout: Causes and Cure.* New York, NY: The Free Press.

Popay J. 2006. *Moving Beyond Effectiveness: Methodological Issues in the Synthesis of Diverse Sources of Evidence.* London: National Institute for Health and Clinical Excellence.

Porter M. E. 1985. *Competitive Advantage: Creating and Sustaining Superior Performance.* New York, NY: The Free Press.

Porter M. E. 2011. *What is Value in Health Care?* Cambridge, MA: Harvard Business School, Institute for Strategy and Competitiveness.

Putnam, H. 2002. *The Collapse of the Fact/Value Dichotomy and Other Essays.* Cambridge, MA: Harvard University Press.

QIPP Right Care. 2010, *Reducing Unwarranted Variation to Increase Value and Improve Quality.* London: Department of Health.

QIPP Right Care. 2011. *Commissioning for Value: Outline programme for 2011/12.* NHS Right Care programme. London: Department of Health.

QIPP Workstreams. 2011. *End of Life QIPP.* London: Department of Health.

Quinn, R. E. and Rohrbaugh, J. 1983. A spatial model of effectiveness criteria: towards a competing values approach to organizational analysis. *Management Science* 29, 363–377.

Rawls J. 1971. *A Theory of Justice,* revised ed. London: Belknap Press.

Rawls J. 1999. *A Theory of Justice,* second edition. Cambridge, MA: Harvard University Press.

Reed S. 2011. Cooperative Council launched. Available at: http://cllrstevereed.wordpress.com/.

Roberts T., Bryan S., Heginbotham C. and McCallum A. 2001. Public involvement in health care priority setting: an economic perspective. *Health Expectations* 2(4), 235–244.

Robinson N. 1999. The use of focus group methodology – with selected examples from sexual health research. *Journal of Advanced Nursing* 29(4), 905–913.

Rother, M. and Shook, J. 2003. *Learning to See: Value Stream Mapping to Create Value and Eliminate Muda.* Cambridge, MA: Lean Enterprise Institute Inc.

Royal College of Psychiatrists. 2010. *No Health Without Public Mental Health: The Case for Action.* London: Royal College of Psychiatrists.

Rubin J. B. 2007. Psychoanalysis and spirituality. *In: Psychoanalysis and religion in the 21st Century,* reprint edition, Black D M, ed. London: Routledge, pp. 132–153.

Sabat S. R. 2011. *The Experience of Alzheimers Disease: Life Through a Tangled Veil.* Oxford: Blackwell.

Sackett D. L. 1997. Evidence based medicine. *Seminars in Perinatology* 21(1), 3–5.

Sackett D. L., Staus S. E., Scott Richardson W. and Haynes R. B. 2000. *Evidence-Based Medicine: How to Practice and Teach EBM.* Edinburgh: Churchill Livingstone.

Sadler J. Z. 2004. *Values and Psychiatric Diagnosis.* Oxford: Oxford University Press.

Schneiderman, L. J. 2011. Defining medical futility and improving medical care. *Journal of Bioethical Inquiry* 8(2):123–131.

Schulze B. and Angermeyer C. 2003. Subjective experiences of stigma. A focus group study of schizophrenic patients, their relatives and mental health professionals. *Social Science & Medicine* 56(2), 299–312.

Seedhouse, D. 2005. *Values-based Decision-making for the Caring Professions.* Chichester: Wiley.

Sell S. 2010. Fundholding could save £1bn each year, says think tank. *GP.*

Sen A. 2002. *Rationality and Freedom.* Cambrige, MA: Belknap/Harvard.

Sen, A. 2009. *The Idea of Justice.* Cambridge, MA: Belknap/Harvard.

Senge P. M. 1990. *The Fifth Discipline: The Art and Practice of the Learning Organisation.* New York, NY: Currency.

Senge P. M. 1999. *The Dance of Change: The Challenges of Sustaining Momentum in Learning Organisations.* New York, NY: Currency/Doubleday.

Seror R., Tubach F., Baron G., Guillemin F. and Ravaudi P. 2010. Extended report: Measure of function in rheumatoid arthritis: individualised or classical scales? *Annals of the Rheumatic Diseases* 69, 97–101.

Social Enterprise Coalition. 2011. *Social Enterprise Explained.* London: Social Enterprise Coalition.

Social Enterprise Coalition and Hempsons Solicitors. 2007. *Healthy Business – A Guide to Social Enterprise in Health and Social Care*. London: Social Enterprise Coalition and Hempsons Ltd.

Taylor M. 2011. The big idea: councils must be ingenious not innovative. Making the most of the resources you have is the key to redesigning services – and that goes for local government too. *Guardian Professional*.

The Centre for Welfare Reform. 2011. Community Assets. Available at: http://www.centreforwelfarereform.org/innovations/total-place-commissioning.html.

Thistlethwaite P. 2011. *Integrated Working: A Guide*. London: Integrated Care Network.

Treacy M. and Wiersema F. 1995. *The Discipline of Market Leaders: Choose Your Customers, Narrow Your Focus, Dominate Your Market*. New York, NY: HarperCollins.

Turning Point with Dr. Foster. 2011. *A Personal Approach to Public Services*. London, Author.

Ulwick A. W. 2002. *Turn Customer Input into Innovation*. New Haven, CT: Harvard Business Review.

van Assen, M., den Berg, G. V. and Pietersma, P. 2009. *Key Management Models*, 2nd edition. London: Pearson Education Limited.

Wakefield A. J., Murch S. H., Anthony A., *et al*. 1998. Ileal-lymphoid-nodular hyperplasia, non-specific colitis, and pervasive developmental disorder in children *RETRACTED*. *The Lancet* **351** (9103).

Walker N. 2008. Practical Solutions to Integrating Services. Powerpoint presentation for CSIP (the Care Services Improvement Partnership).

Wanless D. 2004. *Securing Good Health for the Whole Population: Final Report*. London: HM Treasury.

Wennberg J. E., Bronlee S., Fisher E., Skinner J. and Weinstein J. 2008. *An Agenda for Change. Improving Quality and Curbing Health Care Spending: Opportunities for the Congress and the Obama Administration*. Dartmouth, NH: Dartmouth Atlas of Health Care website.

Wilkinson R. and Pickett K. 2009. *The Spirit Level*. London: Allen Lane.

Williams R. 2000. *Lost Icons: Reflections on Cultural Bereavement*. Edinburgh: T&T Clark.

Wood N. and Curry J. 2009. *PBC Two Years On: Moving Forward and Making a Difference?* London: Kings Fund.

Woodbridge K. and Fulford K. W. M. 2004. *Whose Values? A Workbook for Values-based Practice in Mental Health Care*. London: Sainsbury Centre for Mental Health.

World Bank. 1993. *World Bank Development Report*. Washington, DC: World Bank.

Zeeman E. C. 1977. *Catastrophe Theory, Selected Papers*. London: Addison-Wesley.

Zuboff, S. and Maxmin, J. 2003. *The Support Economy: Why Corporations Are Failing Individuals and the Next Episode of Capitalism*. New York, NY: Allen Lane/Penguin.

Index